YOGA AND VITALITY

YOGA AND VITALITY

by

JAMES HEWITT

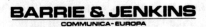
BARRIE & JENKINS
COMMUNICA-EUROPA

© 1977 James Hewitt

First published in 1977 by
Barrie & Jenkins Limited
24 Highbury Crescent, London N5 1RX

ISBN 0 214 20466 9   PAPERBACK
ISBN 0 214 20450 2   HARDBACK

Typeset in Monotype Ehrhardt Series 453 & 573 by Jetset Typesetters Limited
Printed in Great Britain at the Alden Press, Oxford
and bound by Kemp Hall Bindery

Contents

Illustrations

The line drawings of postures are by Ted Ripley.
The Indian illustrations are from the Richard
von Garbe Collection published in Richard
Schmidt's *Fakire und Fakirtum in alten und
modernen Indien* (Berlin, 1908).

Preface

The philosophical, metaphysical, and religious bases of Yoga may be accepted or denied, in whole or in part; but there can be no gainsaying the rewards of greater health, vitality, and psycho-physical poise that result from Yoga practice, as many thousands of men and women have discovered recently in the West. In the East yoga has been practised for thousands of years. Only in this century has it been introduced into Europe and America, but it is now firmly established. It has proved to be no passing fad, simply because it fulfils its promises, supplying the results expected of it at whichever level it is practised.

It is on the *practice* of Yoga, and also on the *practical* in Yoga, that I have concentrated in writing *Yoga and Vitality*, and in writing two complementary works, *Yoga Postures* and *Yoga and Meditation*. The three volumes together comprise what is virtually an encyclopedia of Yoga practice and of practical Yoga. This practical approach is aimed at enriching the health and consciousness of people going about the complicated, stress-beset activity of present-day living. Yoga has always provided for the needs of 'householder Yogins' – men and women practising Yoga without withdrawing from family life and responsibilities.

In making a practical approach to Yoga we satisfy the demands of students who consider the rewards of psycho-physical health and poise worthy aims in themselves. We also provide the aspirant who wishes for 'higher consciousness' and mystical experience with the groundwork which equips him for the climb. The analogy with mountain climbing is apt for the postures, breath controls, cleansing processes, and healthful eating habits and diet of physiological Yoga, called Hatha Yoga, prepare the aspirant for the subtle disciplines of psychical Yoga, called Raja Yoga. Raja Yoga refines consciousness and aims at the pinnacle of intuitive enlightenment (*samadhi*).

The three volumes are concerned mainly with these two Yogas, Hatha and Raja – the Yogas most widely practised in the West and most easily adaptable to occidental needs.

Yoga and Vitality is intended to establish the student securely in Yogic practice; to raise levels of health, energy, and psycho-physical poise, through control of breathing, posture, hygiene, relaxation, and diet. Breath control (*pranayama*) is at the heart of the Yoga of vitality. It has been neglected in much of the literature of Yoga for Westerners, but in this book it is given the emphasis it deserves. An example of our direct and practical approach is that the *bandhas* and *mudras* of Hatha Yoga, which are special postures and muscle controls, are employed not for prolonged breath suspension and the arousal of mysterious energies, but for the enhancement of sexual health and fitness. *Yoga and Vitality* also includes a balanced programme of general postures.

Yoga Postures presents by far the largest collection of postures (*asanas*) ever published – over 400. They include warm-up and limber-up exercises, which most Western students need before embarking on a programme of posturing; and modifications and simplifications of postures which can lead to full performance of the classic *asanas*. Thus there are programmes to suit any stage of suppleness.

Yoga and Meditation describes the most direct and practical techniques of meditation, including the traditional method of *Patanjali*, the transcendental meditation of Maharishi Mahesh Yogi, and recent Western experiments in auto-control of the involuntary nervous system using electrical biofeedback apparatus.

Each of the three volumes – *Yoga and Vitality*, *Yoga Postures*, and *Yoga and Meditation* – stands on its own, but the three combine to make a clear and practical guide for practitioners of Yoga who wish to garner its many benefits for body and mind, and to improve the whole quality of everyday life. For Yoga is a life-science and a life-style.

Finally, a point concerning the printing of this book and of the two complementary volumes: I have followed the practice of many works written on Yoga for a mainly Western readership by omitting diacritical marks in the printing of words in Sanskrit, the classic language of Indian Yoga.

JAMES HEWITT

I Yoga and Yogas

WHAT IS YOGA?

Confusion will be avoided if we at once point out that there is Yoga as an end-goal and Yoga as a system of techniques and disciplines to reach the end-goal. Not only that: there are several systems, and therefore several Yogas. But the aim in each case is the same, though it is talked about in the language of a variety of religions and cultures. Strictly speaking, Yoga is Indian and Hindu; and for the Hindu mystic the supreme goal in living is absorption in *Brahman* – 'I am that.'

Who or what is *Brahman*? In the purest Yoga, which is that of the *upanishads*, *Brahman* is impersonal and imageless, and should not be confused with Brahma, a deity of the Hindu Trinity (the other members are Siva and Vishnu). *Brahman* as the One of world mysticism can be written about in a variety of ways, not all of them religious. Mysticism does not belong solely to the world religions, though it is linked closely with them. How does one classify Buddhism, which has no god, and looks on its founder, at a sophisticated level, as an enlightened man? Each age and culture finds its appropriate vocabulary for the One. In the West today, a psychological orientation makes Being, Self beyond empirical ego, and levels of consciousness the terms in which the loftiest aims of Yoga are most meaningfully discussed.

The Self to be realized beyond the ego in Indian Yoga is the *Atman*. Find the *Atman*, which is pure consciousness, through Yogic practice, and you find (the intuitive enlightenment called *samadhi*) that individual being and Cosmic Being have the same ground, and that *Atman* and *Brahman* are one. This realized union is called Yoga – the word comes from roots meaning 'union', and, the English 'yoke' is etymologically related.

A Yoga is also a system of physical and psychical controls whose aim is to make the practitioner aware of the identity of *Atman* and *Brahman*, or the ground of Being, or whatever concepts are found congenial. And even if you remain agnostic or sceptical towards the whole mystic concept, there remains such value in the bodily exercises and meditative techniques in terms of psycho-physical well-being that thousands of people practise Yoga with barely a thought for Yoga as a mystical goal. Their concern is with Yoga as practice.

THE SVETASVATARA UPANISHAD

The above points become clearer if we look at a concise description of Yoga practice and its powers found in the *Svetasvatara Upanishad*, II, 8–15 (114)

> If a wise man hold his body with its three erect parts (chest, neck, and head) even, and turn his senses with the mind towards the heart, he will then in the boat of *Brahman* cross all the torrents which cause fear.
>
> Compressing his breathings let him who has subdued all motions, breathe forth through the nose with gentle breath. Let the wise man without fail restrain his mind, that chariot yoked with vicious horses.
>
> Let him perform his exercises in a place level, pure, free from pebbles, fire, and dust, delightful by its sounds, its water, and bowers, not painful to the eye, and full of shelters and caves.
>
> When Yoga is being performed, the forms which come first, producing apparitions in *Brahman*, are those of misty smoke, sun, fire, wind, fire-flies, lightnings, and a crystal moon.
>
> When, as earth, water, light, heat, and ether arise, the fivefold quality of Yoga takes place, then there is no longer illness, old age, or pain for him who has obtained a body, produced by the fire of Yoga.
>
> The first results of Yoga they call lightness, healthiness, steadiness, a good complexion, an easy pronunciation, a sweet odour, and slight excretions.
>
> As a metal disk [mirror], tarnished by dust, shines bright again after it has been cleaned, so is the one incarnate person satisfied and free from grief, after he has seen the real nature of the self.
>
> And when by means of the real nature of his self he sees, as by a

lamp, the real nature of *Brahman*, then having known the unborn, eternal god, who is beyond all natures, he is freed from all fetters.

In the above quotation we see Yoga as goal (absorption in *Brahman*); Yoga as postures and breath controls; and Yoga as meditation and contemplation. The two most widely practised Yogas in the West are here indicated: the physiological Yoga, called Hatha Yoga, and the Yoga of mental mastery, called Raja Yoga. We will sometimes refer to them as the Yoga of Vitality and the Yoga of Meditation respectively. The Yoga of Posture is part of Hatha Yoga, or the Yoga of Vitality.

CLASSIFYING THE YOGAS

When it comes to classifying and grouping the systems of Yoga, one finds differences of opinion among the scholars. The reason for this is that the Yogas overlap and interpenetrate to such an extent that several classifications have validity. It is possible to use a system that incorporates several Yogas directly, and several others indirectly. And some people attempt nothing less than a synthesis of all the main Yogas. Swami Vivekananda and Sri Aurobindo have expounded this approach eloquently in their writings.

In *Yoga and Vitality* we will be describing methods taken from Hatha Yoga, which some people do not consider a Yoga at all, but a system of exercises that can serve other Yogas. But the main tradition sees it as purificatory preparation for Raja (Royal) Yoga. Hatha Yoga is the most widely practised Yoga in the West: it includes the well-known postures and breath controls.

The Yogas other than Hatha are mainly meditative and more directly aimed at Yoga as end-goal and union. Their practices will appear later in *Yoga and Meditation*. For the present it is sufficient to name them and indicate their nature briefly. However, even in performing the physical techniques of Hatha Yoga, to some extent one cannot avoid practising other Yogas.

At this stage the main Indian Yogas may be discerned as follows:

Jnana Yoga	Union by knowledge
Bhakti Yoga	Union by love and devotion
Karma Yoga	Union by action and service
Mantra Yoga	Union by voice and sound

Yantra Yoga	Union by vision and form
Laya and Kundalini Yoga	Union by arousal of latent psychic nerve-force
Tantric Yoga	A general term for the physiological disciplines. Also union by harnessing sexual energy
Hatha Yoga	Union by bodily mastery (principally of breath)
Raja Yoga	Union by mental mastery

Jnana Yoga

This is the path of spiritual knowledge and wisdom, suited to the intellectual temperament, in which the intellect penetrates the veils of ignorance that prevent man from seeing his True Self (*Atman*), which is other than the empirical ego. The disciplines of this path of the well-honed intellect are those of study and meditation.

Bhakti Yoga

This is the Yoga of strongly-focused love, devotion, and worship, at its finest in love of the One. The Hindu may concentrate his devotion upon a worshipped deity (Krishna is the most popular) or upon the divine principle as incarnated in a *guru*. Bhakti Yoga is accessible to Westerners with highly devotional temperaments; others are made to feel uncomfortable by some of the excesses. This could be said to be the favourite Yoga of the Indian masses. Its disciplines are those of rites and the singing of songs of praise. St Francis of Assisi is often mentioned as an example of a Christian *bhakti*.

Karma Yoga

This is the path of selfless action and service, without thought of the fruits of action. Its most eloquent exposition is the Lord Krishna's instruction of the young prince Arjuna in the *Bhagavad Gita*. Mahatma Gandhi, the father of modern India, could be looked on as a Karma Yogin.

Mantra Yoga

The practice of Mantra Yoga influences consciousness through repeating (aloud or inwardly) certain syllables, words, or phrases (*mantras*). A form of Mantra Yoga is being practised by many thousands of Westerners, in the form of the Transcendental Meditation taught by Maharishi Mahesh Yogi. Rhythmic repetition of *mantras* is called *japa*. The most highly-regarded *mantras* are 'OM' and 'OM MANE PADME HUM'.

Yantra Yoga

As Mantra Yoga influences consciousness through the vibrations of the voice and sound, so Yantra Yoga employs sight and form. The colourful *mandalas* of Northern India and Tibet are objects of contemplation to Yogins. The visualization may be with the inner eye, just as listening to a *mantra* may be with the inner ear. A *yantra* is a design with power to influence consciousness: it can be an objective picture, an inner visualization, or the design of a temple.

Laya and Kundalini Yoga

These combine many of the techniques of Hatha Yoga, especially prolonged breath suspension and a stable posture, with intense meditative concentration, so as to awaken the psychic nerve-force latent in the body, symbolized as serpent power (*kundalini*), which is coiled below the base of the spine. The force is taken up the spine, passing through several power centres (*chakras*), until it reaches a *chakra* in the crown of the head, when intuitive enlightenment (*samadhi*) is triggered. The physiological and concentrative disciplines are severe, and this is a Yoga best practised with personal supervision by a teacher.

Tantric Yoga

'Tantric' is applied as a general term to distinguish physiological systems from those that are non-physiological. Tantrism is also a form of Yoga, found mainly in Northern India and Tibet, in which control of the sexual energies has a prominent part, and the union of male and female (Yogi and Yogini), either actually or in an act of imaginative creation, has a ritualistic role. Tantric Yoga, of all the Yogas, guards its teachings and techniques most closely. This sexual Yoga may be looked upon with a measure of disapproval by adherents of some of the other schools.

Hatha Yoga

The word Hatha derives from two roots: *ha* means 'sun' and *tha* means 'moon'. The flow of breath in the right nostril is called the 'sun breath' and the flow of breath in the left nostril is the 'moon breath'. Central to all Hatha Yoga disciplines is the regulation of breath, the harmonizing of its positive (sun) and negative (moon), or male and female currents. Another meaning of the word Hatha is 'forced', but the term Forced Yoga would not do justice to the poised and gentle nature of most Yogic controls.

This is the Yoga best known and most widely practised in the West, and the subject of the majority of popular manuals on Yoga. Its best-known feature is posturing – in particular sitting with the legs crossed and the feet upturned on the thighs (Lotus Posture or *Padmasana*) and standing on the head (Headstand Posture or *Sirsasana*). *Asana*, which now means a Yogic posture, originally meant 'seat' or 'sitting method', an indication that the wide range of postures developed from a few basic positions for sitting in meditation.

Hatha Yoga exercises are practised extensively in the West for their practical benefits to the health of the nervous system, glands, and vital organs. When it is practised similarly in India it is sometimes called Ghatastha Yoga; but there physiological Yoga is less often separated from its over-all mystical setting and purpose.

Hatha Yoga may be viewed as a hygiene which takes into account the purification of the total organism. It may sound quotidian to some people to call this Yoga a hygiene, but there is a mainstream tradition that sees Hatha Yoga as a purificatory preparation for Raja Yoga, which is work upon consciousness itself. Such mental disciplining can best be effected in a healthy, relaxed body in which the energies have been equalized.

The French writer C. Kerneiz, writing under the pseudonym 'Felix Guyot', opened his book *Yoga : the Science of Health* (35) with these words:

> Keep well, remain young a long time, and live to a good old age, such is the threefold wish that the men of every race and country have, at all times, formulated at the bottom of their hearts. This threefold wish is a very natural one, for it is simply the expression of the most powerful and the most tenacious of instincts: self-preservation. Live! We want to live with the greatest amplitude possible.
>
> To fight against disease, when it comes, and to avert, as far as is possible, the threat of death which is in its train; to defer old age, and, by doing so, put off death itself, we have hygiene, which is only, it is

true, an autonomous but not independent province of the medical kingdom.

But there exists a science, practised in India and Tibet, and more or less throughout the whole of China, which is somewhat mysterious, for it is not taught to all comers. This science is traditional and its origin is lost in the night of time. It has precisely the same object as hygiene in Western countries: to keep its adepts in health and strength and to ward off old age and death for the longest time possible. This science of Life, which is only a branch of the secret of the Yogis, is called the Hatha Yoga.

Raja Yoga

Hatha Yoga is the most practical of Yogas, with its emphasis on promoting vibrant health and tapping the organism's latent energies. It has, too, an integrating and calming influence on the mind. But the direct work of mastering consciousness and stilling thought so as to become aware of the Ground of Being belongs to Raja or Royal Yoga. Raja Yoga is considered royal because the Yogin who practises this Yoga thereby becomes ruler over his mind.

Raja Yoga is closely associated with the systematization of Yoga techniques by Patanjali (who lived about the third or second century BC) in his *Yoga Sutras*. He lists *asanas* (postures) and *pranayama* (breath controls) among his 'eight limbs' of Yoga, and such classic texts as the *Hatha Yoga Pradipika*, the *Gheranda Samhita*, and the *Siva Samhita* follow Patanjali in seeing Hatha Yoga practices as providing a physiological hygiene that prepares the body for effective mental control. According to this view, Raja Yoga includes Hatha Yoga within its system.

Hatha Yoga works upon the body, purifying and perfecting it, and through the body upon the mind. Raja Yoga works upon the mind, refining and perfecting it, and through the mind upon the body. But just as some people practise the physiological Yogas with little or no thought for mental disciplines, so there are exponents of the mental Yogas who consider that the body will respond beneficially to control of consciousness without having to resort to anything more 'physical' than a stable posture in sitting for meditation. But a great number of Yogins combine the physiological Yoga of Vitality with the psychical Yoga of Meditation.

OVERLAPPING OF PATHS

From examination of the brief summary of the main Yoga systems just given, you will perceive that it would be difficult to practise any one of them without to some extent incorporating elements from others. Concentration, a central feature of Raja Yoga, operates in all the other paths in varying degrees. The devotion of Bhakti Yoga provides some motive power and affective feeling tone in performing the actions of Karma Yoga, the exercises of Hatha Yoga, the incantations of Mantra Yoga, the visualizations of Yantra Yoga, and so on – even the intellectual work of Jnana Yoga is not without this affective colouring. One could trace at some length this criss-crossing of Yoga paths.

THE CLASSIC TEXTS OF HATHA YOGA

The three main classic treatises on Hatha Yoga are the *Hatha Yoga Pradipika* ('Light on the Hatha Yoga'), the *Gheranda Samhita* ('Gheranda's Compendium'), and the *Siva Samhita* ('Siva's Compendium'). The first-named is considered to be the standard work.

These texts – like Patanjali's guide to Raja Yoga – were written tersely and in such a way that expansion and elucidation by teachers was required. Until recent times a teacher was essential, but now books (such as this one) can act as instructors in practical Yoga suited to the needs of the majority of men and women who have no desire to withdraw from the customary activities of living in the modern world.

It is hardly surprising that these old texts, representing a tradition older still, should contain much that to modern eyes appears unscientific, superstitious, incomprehensible, magical, bizarre, and outmoded. The language is at times exaggerated, and as with so much of this type of literature, scholars have fun disputing among themselves over what was intended to be taken literally and what symbolically. Much of the instruction today's readers will wish to discard: for example, the injunction to rub the ashes of dried cow's dung on the skin.

SANSKRIT – CLASSIC LANGUAGE OF YOGA

English belongs to an extensive family of languages that includes

most of the languages of Europe and of India, and so is given the
name Indo-European. A subfamily of the Indo-European group is
the Indo-Iranian, or Aryan. The people who spoke these languages
thought so highly of themselves that they called themselves Aryans,
or 'noble ones'. The Aryans seem to have invaded India from the
north-west, from Afghanistan or Iran. The oral tradition of their
ancient Vedic hymns in time gave way to a form of language called
Sanskrit, and this was standardized about 300 BC. It is the language
of the sacred texts of Hinduism and the classic texts of Yoga. Its
place in Indian learning could be said to correspond to that of Latin
in Europe.

The relationship between English, Latin, Greek, and Sanskrit
can be gathered from these few examples:

Mod. Eng.	Old Eng.	Gothic	Latin	Greek	Sanskrit
Father	Fnder	Fadar	Pater	Pater	Pitar
Three	Thrie	—	Tres	Treis	Trayas
Six	Siex	Saihs	Sex	Hex	Sas
Nine	Nigon	Niun	Novem	Ennea	Nava

Sanskrit words abound in Yogic literature – the many postures
(*asanas*), for example, have Sanskrit names. But English speakers
should restrict their use of Sanskrit to the written word: otherwise
they may receive a nasty shock one day on hearing a native Indian
pronounce the Yogic terms correctly.

BENEFITS FROM THE YOGA OF VITALITY

Mr Archie J. Bahm, in his book *Yoga for Business Executives* (5),
devotes no less than sixty-two pages to discussing the immediate,
long-range, and comparative values of Yoga. Not even a summary
of the benefits will be offered here. They are touched upon here and
there in this book, and will be detailed further in dealing with each
group of controls and exercises. It may have been necessary a few
years ago to 'sell' Hatha Yoga, but it is not necessary now. The West
has got the message – *Yoga works*.

This book will tell the reader what it is that Yoga asks him to
do – in a word, *practice*. As the *Hatha Yoga Pradipika* (75) says:
Whether young, old or too old, sick or lean, one who discards laziness,
gets success if he practises Yoga. Success comes to him who is engaged

in the practice; for by merely reading books on Yoga, one can never get success. Success cannot be attained by adopting a particular dress. It cannot be gained by telling tales. Practice alone is the means of success.

II Yogic Relaxation

CORPSE POSTURE (*Savasana*)

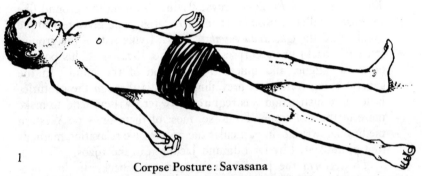

1

Corpse Posture: Savasana
The Yogin's head, shoulders, back, buttocks, leg and feet must rest on
the ground in this posture of relaxation.

All techniques of Yoga aim to produce tranquillity. Postures, breath
controls, mind-stilling meditation, the bodily, mental, and spiritual
purifications – all have a relaxing influence that is widely
acknowledged as probably Yoga's greatest advantage for Western
man. For he lives at a pace unknown to his forefathers and his
nervous system has to cope with a bombardment of stimuli that
would have been intolerable to earlier generations. Those who
embrace Yoga practice in its full range – that is, Yoga of Vitality,
Yoga of Posture, and Yoga of Meditation – will achieve the maximum body-mind harmony and relaxation. But even those men and
women who practise only the postures, perhaps at evening classes
or at home, report: 'I am more relaxed,' 'My emotions are under
control,' 'My nerves are calm,' or 'I feel more tranquil.' This
frequently is acknowledged after only a few weeks of Yoga practice.

Among the postures are several which aim directly at relaxation. Here we will describe only one – but far and away the most important: the strangely-named Corpse Posture (*Savasana* or *Mrtasana*). It is customary to spend a few minutes 'playing dead' in this posture immediately before and immediately after a programme of *asanas*. Readers fully involved in the hurly-burly of modern civilized living should ensure that a few minutes relaxation are taken in this pose each day, because of its great restorative powers.

HOW TO RELAX

The *Hatha Yoga Pradipika* says: 'Lying down on the ground like a corpse is called *Savasana*. It removes fatigue and gives rest to the mind.' And the *Gheranda Samhita* says: 'Lying flat on the ground (on one's back) like a corpse is called the *Mrtasana*. This posture destroys fatigue, and quiets the agitation of the mind.' In the general living conditions prevailing in India through the centuries little more instruction was required. Western writers tend to make more of the technique. To do so, most of them draw on Western medical knowledge, in particular the progressive relaxation methods first promulgated by Dr Edmund Jacobson in the 1920s.

To perform the posture, lie flat on your back, the legs outstretched so that the heels are a little apart and the feet have fallen limply outwards. The arms lie alongside the body, resting on the floor, the palms of the hands turned up, with the fingers limp and slightly curled. Thin cushions may be placed below the neck and each knee.

Now observe your breathing, which should be through the nostrils, not the mouth. Do not interfere with the in-and-out flow of the breath: just observe. Take two successive deep abdominal breaths, fully exhaling. The abdomen swells out on the inhalation and draws back towards the spine on the exhalation. Then let go with the abdominal muscles and return to observing the rise and fall of respiration. Soon you will notice that your breathing has become quiet, smooth, and of even rhythm. Occasionally during relaxation you may experience an involuntary deep intake of breath, followed by a sighing exhalation. This should be welcomed as a sign that tension is being dissolved somewhere in the musculature.

Having established your breathing in a quiet, smooth, and rhythmic pattern, you next employ your attention like a torch beam to play over your body from feet to scalp, looking for tension, and letting go from it. Relaxation is a letting go from tension. The postures and breathing exercises of Yoga will help to put you on intimate speaking terms with your body muscles in a way you are unlikely to have experienced since childhood. Look upon the various sections of your body listed below as listening muscles ready to obey your silently spoken command – which is simply two words: 'let go.' As a muscle or muscle group lets go, you should instantly feel it become heavier: like the sleeping baby or cat, it rests with its full weight. Think of tension draining away like a dangerous poison from the muscles and body parts listed below. Note carefully the feeling of relaxation.

STAGE BY STAGE RELAXATION

Stage by stage, the relaxation sequence is as follows:
   i.   Lie flat on your back in the Corpse Posture.
   ii.   Observe your breathing, without seeking to control it, for a few minutes.
   iii.   Make two successive deep inhalations and exhalations, swelling out the abdomen on breathing in and drawing it in towards the backbone on breathing out. Relax the abdominal wall fully at the conclusion of the second breath.
   iv.   Observe your breathing again. When it has become quiet, smooth, and of even rhythm, direct your attention like a torch beam in sequence over the parts of the body listed below. Look for tension in each part and let go from it, so that the muscles rest with their full weight. Note carefully the sensations of tension, then of absence of tension (relaxation). The sequence is: left foot; left calf; left thigh, front and rear; right foot; right calf; right thigh, front and rear; pelvis; abdomen; lower back; chest; upper back; left hand; left forearm; left upper arm, front and rear; left shoulder; right hand; right forearm; right upper arm, front and rear; right shoulder; throat; neck; jaw; lips; tongue; eyes; brow; scalp. In relaxing the feet and hands, do not forget the toes and fingers, each one of which should be drained of tension and feel limp.
   v.   Observe your breathing again for a minute or two; then

repeat the sequence of letting go with the muscles from feet to scalp.
Continue in the manner just described for as many minutes as you
are giving to relaxation. Fifteen to thirty minutes is a good average.

At the conclusion of each wave of relaxation from feet to scalp,
the whole body should rest with its full weight and feel drained of
tension. The mind also should be at peace.

RELAXING THE FACIAL MUSCLES

In view of the importance of relaxing the facial muscles, I suggest
a few aids that will be found effective:

To help relax the jaw: yawn slowly, resisting evenly all the way
with the muscles of the jaw. Hold the contraction for six seconds;
then let go, close the mouth, and let the jaw sag.

To help relax the lips: purse and push forward the lips as though
to kiss, taking note of the sensations of tension. Hold the kiss
position for six seconds; then relax the lips fully.

To help relax the tongue: keeping the teeth together, touch the
roof of the mouth as far back as you can with the tip of the tongue.
Keep the tongue immobile in that position for six seconds; then let
go fully, so that the tongue 'floats' in the mouth with its tip behind
the lower teeth.

To help relax the eyes: without moving the head, look as far to
the left as possible; as far to the right as possible; as far upwards as
possible; as far downwards as possible. Thinking of this in terms of
the Clock Exercise, you look at nine o'clock; three o'clock; twelve
o'clock; and six o'clock. Take note throughout of the sensations of
tension in the muscles that move the eyeballs; then give equal
attention to the feeling of relaxation as you let go and close your eyes.

To help relax the brow: frown strongly, contracting the muscles
of the brow. Hold the contraction for six seconds; then let go fully.
This is a useful technique to combat worry, which registers in
forehead tensions.

To help relax the scalp: without moving your head, move the
scalp forwards and backwards a few times by conscious control.
Then let go fully with the scalp muscles.

AIDS TO RELAXATION

Many imaginative techniques are suggested by writers on Yoga to aid relaxation in the Corpse Posture. One idea is to imagine that you are lying on a beach, listening to the soothing sound of the sea and feeling the caress of a gentle breeze and warm sunlight on your flesh.

Another suggestion is to imagine a tiny hole in the small of the back from which tension drains away. This has the effect of flattening the back along the floor and encourages lying with the full weight.

Yet another imaginative technique could be described as the Water Method. You think of a current of water slowly flowing through the body, cleansing it of all tensions and impurities. You think of it flowing through the neck, in the shoulders and along the arms, into the chest, on to the abdomen, down the spine, through the buttocks, filling the thighs, knees, calves, and feet. Finally the purifying water – which is best thought of as warm – trickles away from the fingers and toes. This can be imagined as happening several times.

As skill in relaxation develops, you will find that you are able to let go from tension in sitting as well as in supine positions.

All Yogic practice counters stress, recognized by doctors as one of the greatest threats to health and life faced by modern man. So the Corpse Posture, being specifically intended for relaxation, should not be neglected by any Western practitioner who wishes to protect himself (or herself) from this contemporary killer.

III Yogic Posturing

THE YOGI AS A FREAK

During the winter of 1896-7 Bava Luchman Dass, a Punjabi, described as 'a Brahmin of the highest caste,' performed the postures or *asanas* of Hatha Yoga in a side-show at the Westminster Aquarium in London, giving between sixty and seventy performances a day for forty days. Outside the show was displayed a framed cheque for £500 'which anyone can claim who emulates the Yoga's [*sic*] fearful and wonderful contortions.'

The performances evoked merriment and humorous comment from the paying viewers. When the Yogi adopted a Kneeling Lotus Posture, a Cockney voice remarked: 'It's a fine mode of pedomotion for a man cursed with corns.' Reporters from newspapers and magazines quoted such remarks, and had their own more sophisticated fun in commenting on the Brahmin's 'contortions,' his diet of goat's milk and dried fruit, and his strange appearance – he was dressed in a woolly leotard and large baggy drawers to meet the requirements of Victorian modesty.

If the Yogin had been a yeti, he could not have occasioned more astonishment or rude and ignorant comment from the general public and journalists alike. No understanding was shown of the lofty aims of Yoga or of the significance of the postures so expertly performed (there is the evidence of photographs) by the unfortunate Punjabi. Unfortunate, because he had been brought to England under false pretences. Thinking he was to demonstrate the ancient art and science of Hatha Yoga exercise, held in almost sacred regard in his own country, to leading citizens of London who might have an interest in perfecting body, mind, and spirit, he found himself stranded in a foreign city, thousands of miles from his homeland, and being *exhibited as a freak*.

The editor of the *Strand Magazine*, (117), who adopted a humorous style in a report of the Yogi's performance, observed:
> From what I gathered, I came to the conclusion that when the ghastly consciousness that he was a side-show dawned upon the Yoga [*sic*], he didn't like it at all, and nothing would induce him to go through his sixty or seventy performances a day but the near prospect of a return to his own native land.

THE CURRENT POPULARITY OF YOGA POSTURING

For today's counterparts of Bava Luchman Dass it is a different story. They can set themselves up as respected teachers of Yoga in London, Paris, Amsterdam, New York, and even the smaller cities in Europe and America, and instruct men and women, drawn from multifarious walks of life, in body control – that same body control which was mocked and occasioned such merriment in the London of 1896–7. Yoga continued to attract more mockery and derision than respect and understanding in Western countries until the rapid acceleration of its acceptance which began in the 1950s. Today there is a waiting list for membership of classes in Yoga posturing. What was once thought by many to be a short-lived craze has been established unshakeably for more than two decades. Only one conclusion can be drawn from this: Yoga posturing is worth doing – it brings worthwhile results.

THE AIMS OF POSTURING

'There is not a single *asana* that is not intended directly or indirectly to quiet the mind,' wrote Dr Theos Bernard, an American who underwent in India the most austere and far-reaching disciplines of Hatha Yoga, which he mastered to a remarkable degree. He continued (7):
> The teacher emphasizes that the primary purpose of the *asanas*, is the reconditioning of the system, both mind and body, so as to effect the highest possible standard of muscular tone, mental health, and organic vigour. Hence stress is put upon the nervous and glandular systems. Hatha Yoga is interpreted as a method that will achieve the maximum

results by the minimum expenditure of energy. The various *asanas* have been devised primarily to stimulate, exercise, and massage the specific areas that demand attention.

A balanced programme of postures works upon every muscle, nerve, gland, and organ in the body. 'Being the first accessory of Hatha Yoga, *asana* is discussed first,' says the *Hatha Yoga Pradipika* (75). 'It should be practised for gaining steady posture, health and lightness of body.' This quotation points out the rewards accurately and succinctly, and is free from the fantastic claims of occult and magical powers found elsewhere in this and other classic texts.

THE UNIQUE CHARACTER OF THE *ASANAS*

You will find nothing like the *asanas* in Western systems of body-culture, and they are also distinct in character from other Eastern exercises. They are not movements, but postures to be adopted and held; most are relaxing rather than effortful, refreshing rather than fatiguing; they are non-competitive; they require no special equipment or clothing; they can be performed by men and women, and persons in all age groups. They take into account the well-being of the whole human organism; their aim is to bring body, mind, and spirit into harmony and equilibrium.

THE ORIGINS OF THE *ASANAS*

Asana is a posture or pose. It is pronounced with the emphasis on the first 'a' – really ā, diacritical marks having been omitted in the printing of this work. The original purpose seems to have been to provide rock-like steadiness in sitting for meditation, for *asana* originally meant 'seat.' The forest sages of old sat immobile for hours, and modern masters do the same. Naturally a compact stable sitting position was needed, in which one would not sway about or fall asleep. A straight back and a low centre of gravity, just below the navel, with unimpaired deep abdominal breathing, were also found to be essential. It looks as though out of this beginning developed a great system of postures, to be held for seconds, minutes, or hours, whose aim was bodily mastery and health. Some *asanas* are çopies of the characteristic movements or poses of the animals, birds, reptiles, and insects after which they are named. The *Surya Namaskars* group (see *Yoga Postures*) would appear to have been originally salutations or prayers to the sun. The term *asana*, which began as the name for one of the sitting postures, is now applied also to standing, supine, prone, and balancing postures.

Yogic postures are depicted in the earliest Indian carvings, and, later, members of the army of Alexander the Great wrote of the gymnastic philosophers they saw in India.

PRE-REQUIREMENTS OF POSTURING

A few commonsense rules should be observed before performing a group of postures. Let at least three hours go by after a main meal, and one hour following a light snack. Empty the bladder, and the bowels too if you can, shortly before exercising. Sponge over the face and body to give a feeling of freshness. Wear loose-fitting clothing, or none at all. Posture in a room that is well-ventilated and free from extremes of temperature. Posture on a firm level floor covered with several thicknesses of blanket.

THE MOST POPULAR CLASSIC *ASANAS*

A study of the now considerable literature of Yogic posturing reveals that of the several hundred Yoga poses, there is a central group of traditional *asanas* held in high regard which can form the base or foundation on which to build varied programmes. We will describe them concisely here, so that a start to posturing can be made without delay; for further development the reader should refer to *Yoga Postures*. Over four hundred postures are described, including the warm-up exercises and the modifications and simplifications of *asanas* that most Western practitioners find essential.

SITTING POSTURES

It is necessary that the student should become acquainted with some of the sitting postures at an early stage. Besides being valuable exercises in themselves, limbering the legs, hips, and pelvis, strengthening the back and improving posture, they provide the sitting position for practising breath control (*pranayama*) and meditation. One cannot start too early learning to sit immobile for several minutes with the back straight and the head poised in line with the spine. The vital energies are gathered and conserved.

The Easy Posture can be adopted immediately by most occidentals; the Egyptian (or Chair) Posture by all. The more difficult sitting postures may take some months to master, but provide maximum seated stability. In these meditative postures the centre of gravity should be felt in the abdomen, a little below the navel. Breathe freely and deeply, using the lower lungs, diaphragm, and abdomen. The postures facilitate deep breathing.

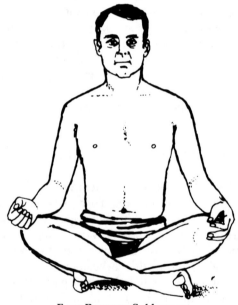

2

Easy Posture: Sukhasana

Easy Posture (Sukhasana)
This is the most practical cross-legged posture for beginners. The ankles are crossed, tailor's fashion, and the knees taken down as low as possible – in time the knees may actually touch the floor. The most important thing is that the head, neck, and spine should be held in a straight vertical line. Vary the ankle crossing, sometimes right over left, sometimes left over right. The right hand should rest

on the right knee and the left hand on the left knee. Breathe freely.

Every opportunity should be taken to sit for several minutes in the Easy Posture – watching television, listening to the radio or records, sewing, feeding baby, and so on.

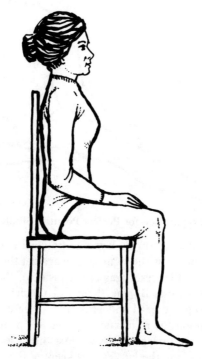

3

Egyptian (or Chair) Posture

Egyptian Posture

Even simpler than the Easy Posture is the Egyptian (or Chair) Posture, but it should only be employed if the Easy Posture proves too uncomfortable.

Sit on a straight-backed chair, the head and spine in vertical line, the feet and knees together, the palm of the right hand flat on the right thigh and the palm of the left hand flat on the left thigh. Breathe freely.

Preparation for Perfect Posture (Siddhasana)

This limbers the ankle, knee, and hip joints for performance of Perfect Posture (*Siddhasana*).

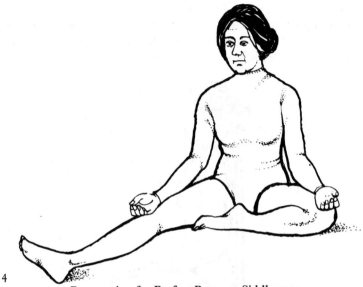

4

Preparation for Perfect Posture: Siddhasana

Sit on the floor with the legs outstretched and well apart. Fold
the right leg and draw the right heel in against the crotch so that the
sole of the right foot rests against the inside of the upper left thigh.
The right knee rests on the floor and the left leg remains fully
extended. Keep the head and back in a straight vertical line. Rest
the right palm on the right knee and the left palm on the left knee.
Breathe freely and deeply. Stay at least thirty seconds in the pose;
then repeat, folding the left leg and keeping the right leg extended.

Perfect Posture (Siddhasana)
Siddha means 'adept' and *siddhas* are 'perfected' Yogins.

As in the preceding Preparation, the right leg is folded and the
heel brought in against the perineum (the soft flesh between genitals
and anus). But this time the left leg is also folded, the left heel is
pulled back against the pubic bone, and the outer edge of the left
foot, sole upturned, is inserted in the fold between the calf and
thigh of the right leg. The thighs and knees of both legs are kept
flat on the floor. Place the right palm on the right knee and the left
palm on the left knee. Sit firmly on the buttocks and legs, keeping
the head and backbone poised in a vertical straight line. Breathe

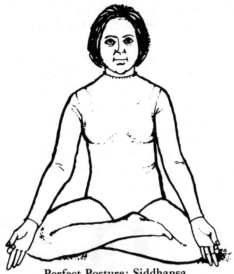

5

Perfect Posture: Siddhansa

freely and deeply. Stay motionless at least one minute; then repeat, reversing the roles of the legs. The pose has great stability and is frequently used for sitting in meditation by master Yogins.

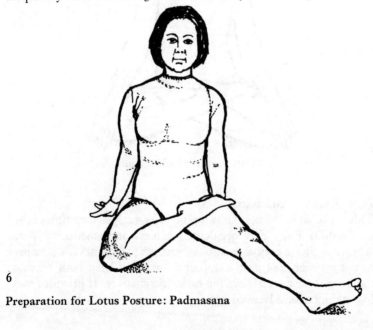

6

Preparation for Lotus Posture: Padmasana

Preparation for Lotus Posture (Padmasana)
Sit on the floor with the legs extended and wide apart. Bend the
right leg at the knee, grasp the right ankle, and pull in the right foot
so that it rests, sole upturned, on top of the left thigh, as high up it
as possible. Keep the back erect and the head in line. Place the
palms of the hands flat on the floor, the left hand beside the left hip
and the right hand beside the right hip. The problem is likely to be
that the right knee is off the floor – gentle pressure from the right
hand may be applied to make the knee lower. After at least thirty
seconds in the pose, during which you should breathe freely and
deeply, straighten the right leg and repeat to the other side, lifting
the left foot on to the right thigh.

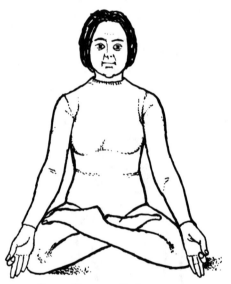

7

Lotus Posture: Padmasana

Lotus Posture (Padmasana)
This is probably the best known pose in Yoga. It is sometimes called
the Buddha Pose. Few occidentals achieve it immediately; some
achieve it after weeks or months of practice; many never do manage
to upturn each foot on the opposite thigh and keep both knees on
the floor. There are always the easier alternatives. It provides rock-
like stability for advanced practice.

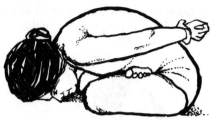

8

Yoga Posture: Yogasana

Yoga Posture (Yogasana)
The Lotus Posture has a role in several advanced postures. We give
one example here. In Yoga Posture you sit in the Lotus Posture,
exhale, bend forward, and lower the forehead to the floor. Stay in
the pose at least twenty seconds, breathing freely. The hands
may be clasped behind the neck or the back.

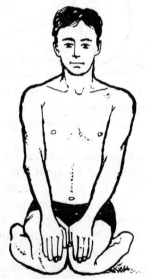

9

Thunderbolt Posture: Vajrasana

Thunderbolt Posture (Vajrasana)
This is worth learning now, for it provides the starting position for
many beneficial postures. It is a favourite sitting position of the
Japanese. Kneel on the floor with the knees together and sit back on
the inner edges of the upturned feet. To do this the toes may be

together, but the heels should be spread apart to support the outer edges of the buttocks. Place the right palm on the right knee and the left palm on the left knee, and keep the head and back erect. Breathe freely and deeply. Stay motionless in the pose for at least one minute.

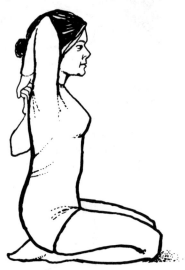

10

Cowface Posture: Gomukhasana

Cowface Posture (Gomukhasana)
This is one of several poses based on the preceding Thunderbolt Posture.

Keep the back erect as you sit on the inner edges of the heels and soles of the feet. Now flex the right arm, raise the right elbow high and lower the right hand down the centre of the back. At the same time bend the left arm and bring the left hand up the spine from below until the fingers of the right hand and those of the left hand hook together. The palm of the right hand faces the back and the palm of the left hand faces outwards. Breathing freely, stay in the pose at least six seconds. Reverse the arm positions and repeat.

If you find that you cannot lock the hands together, hold a handkerchief, towel, or belt so that it is pulled taut, shortening the grip as suppleness increases.

Viewed from the back the pose is said to resemble a cow's face. It improves posture, limbers the shoulder joints, and strengthens and tones the muscles of the shoulders, upper back, and rear upper arms.

A TYPICAL PROGRAMME OF POSTURES

Corpse Posture (Savasana)
First, spend a few minutes lying quietly on the back in the Corpse Posture, fully described in the chapter on Yogic Relaxation. You should commence the programme of postures feeling relaxed and composed. Each of the poses should be given total attention, an essential feature of Yogic posturing.

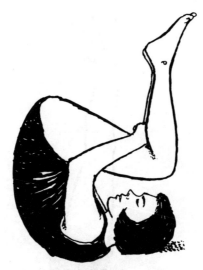

11

Spinal Rock

Spinal Rock
In *Yoga Postures* you will find forty-four warm-up or limber-up exercises, from which several should be selected to prepare the body for the main postures to follow. The muscles and joints benefit greatly from these few preliminary movements. The Indian Yoga masters tend to omit them, but for the majority of occidental students they are important. Many of the warm-ups are valuable exercises in themselves. This could be said of the one selected for inclusion here – the Spinal Rock, also known as the Limbering-up Rock.

Lie flat on the back, bend the legs, and bring the knees together against the chest. The ankles may be together or crossed. Clasp the hands behind the knees or on top of the knees. Now rock gently

forwards and backwards on the rounded back: on the forward rock
the heels should almost touch the floor and on the backward rock
the upper back touches the floor. Breathe in as you rock forward and
breathe out as you rock backward. Continue for at least thirty
seconds.

A useful variation can be added. Rock gently *from side to side* for
at least thirty seconds. This is called the Cradle Rock.

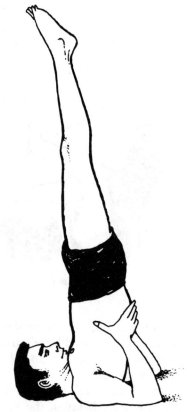

12

Shoulderstand Posture: Sarvangasana

Shoulderstand Posture (Sarvangasana)
The point behind Yoga's inverted poses is that they enable venous
blood to flow easily to the heart, brain, scalp, and facial tissues; at
the same time blood flows out of the legs and lower abdomen, which
tend to become congested. The effect of reversing the normal

directional pull of gravity on the body is refreshing.

The Shoulderstand is suitable for beginners, whereas the full Headstand Posture (*Sirsasana*) needs to be worked up to in stages, as taught in *Yoga Postures*. Even then, the full unsupported Headstand is not for everyone – it is too severe for many persons. The Shoulderstand is the simplest and least strenuous of the inverted poses of Yoga.

Lie flat on the back, the legs outstretched together. Bend the legs and bring the knees backward over the chest. Using the elbows and the backs of the upper arms as props, support the lower back with the palms of the hands, the thumbs outspread. The elbows should not be wider than the shoulders. Now raise the trunk to a vertical position and straighten the legs together so that the trunk and legs form a straight vertical line. The chest is brought against the chin, never the chin to the chest. Breathing freely and deeply, stay steadily in the pose for at least twenty seconds.

The Shoulderstand is unsuitable for persons suffering from high blood pressure or ailments of the neck and head.

Incline-board or Tilt-chair
The benefits of the topsy-turvy poses can be combined with those of relaxation by lying full length on an incline-board placed securely at an angle of thirty-five to forty-five degrees. A sturdy ironing board will serve. For a milder effect one may purchase and use a 'Relaxator' chair, manufactured at West Molesey, Surrey, England, which can be adjusted so as to place the feet higher than the head, at the same time supporting the curvature of the spine in a hammock-type structure. For incline relaxation, follow the stage-by-stage method taught in the chapter on Yogic Relaxation.

Plough Posture (Halasana)
This graceful posture can be performed as an extension of the Shoulderstand. Keeping the legs straight, lower the feet overhead from the Shoulderstand position until the toes rest on the floor. The legs should fall to the floor of their own accord: if they do not at first, they soon will with practice. Breathe freely. This is the Supported Plough Posture. More advanced versions are described in *Yoga Postures*.

This is a superb exercise, stretching the whole body, activating the circulation, and toning the abdomen, hips, and legs. It is said to

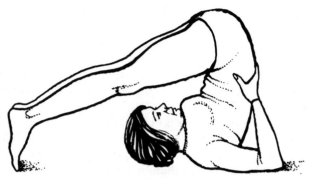

13

Supported Plough Posture: Halasana

improve the health of the endocrine glands, liver, spleen, and
reproductive organs. It is not suitable, however, for persons with
weak vertebrae.

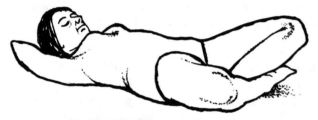

14

Modified Fish Posture: Matsyasana

Fish Posture (Matsyasana)
This is a complementary position to the Plough as the spine is
stretched in the opposite direction. In the advanced version the
legs are crossed and locked in the Lotus position, but the Fish
Posture can also be performed in a simpler version with the ankles
crossed in the Easy Posture.

Lie flat on the back and cross the legs. Keep the knees spread
wide apart and held low to the floor. Now cross the wrists behind
the neck and rest the head on the arms. Breathe deeply into the
abdomen and hold the pose for at least thirty seconds.

In the full version, the legs are crossed in the Lotus position, the
back is arched, and the head is thrown back so that the crown of the
head is on the floor and the shoulders and back are off the floor.
The right hand grasps the left foot and the left hand grasps the
right foot. Breathing freely and deeply, stay in the pose for fifteen

to thirty seconds. The position is a good one for floating easily in water – hence the name Fish Posture.

In this posture the legs and hips are limbered, the thorax is expanded, the pelvis and abdominal viscera are toned, the spine is strengthened, and the spinal nerves are nourished with blood.

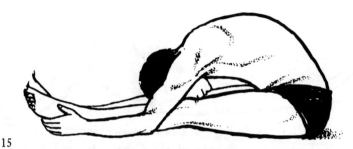

15

Back-stretching Posture: Paschimottanasana

Back-stretching Posture (Paschimottanasana)
Sit on the floor with the legs fully extended together. Take a deep breath; then, exhaling, lower the face towards the knees, at the same time reaching out and down to grasp either the ankles or the feet, as suppleness permits. In advanced practice the face may actually touch the knees and the chest press down on the thighs. Stay down for ten seconds, and then sit up slowly.

The muscles of the back, arms, and legs are stretched, and the spine is stretched and strengthened. The hamstring muscles at the backs of the thighs may protest at first, but they let go and lengthen with practice. The abdomen is massaged as you bend forward, aiding digestion and correcting constipation.

Cobra Posture (Bhujangasana)
Following the Back-stretching Posture, you now turn over and bend the spine in the opposite direction in the Cobra Posture, which resembles a cobra rearing to strike.

Lie full length on the floor, face down, legs together. Bend the arms, keeping the elbows in against the sides, and place the right palm flat on the floor five or six inches in front of the right shoulder (beginners' version) or underneath the shoulder (advanced version). Place the left palm similarly in relation to the left shoulder. In the beginners' version the fingertips are in line horizontally with the chin, which rests on the floor. Inhaling, slowly raise the head, neck,

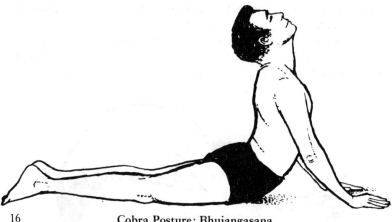

16   **Cobra Posture: Bhujangasana**

and upper back successively, slowly straightening the arms. Rely as
far as possible on the lower back muscles. Hold the pose for at least
ten seconds, the pelvis and legs staying in contact with the floor.
Return slowly to the starting position, exhaling.

The Cobra Posture exercises the spine vertebra by vertebra,
nourishing the spinal nerves with blood. The front of the body is
stretched and the circulation stimulated.

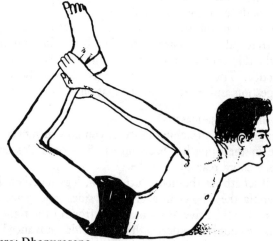

17

Bow Posture: Dhanurasana

Bow Posture (Dhanurasana)
In the Bow Posture the head and trunk are raised up and back as in

the preceding Cobra Posture, but the arms are stretched back so that the right hand grasps the right ankle and the left hand grasps the left ankle. The arms are pulled taut like a bow-string. The beginner will need to spread the knees apart to raise them off the floor; the advanced practitioner brings the knees together. The spine, trunk, and legs take the shape of a bow. Balance on the stomach, breathing freely, for at least six seconds.

In the Bow Posture the whole body is strongly stretched and breathing and circulation are stimulated.

Corpse Posture (Savasana)
Complete the programme, as you began, with a few minutes' relaxation in the Corpse Posture.

PROGRAMME PLANNING

The above short programme is based on some of the most highly regarded Yogic *asanas*, each with a history going back for centuries. The sitting postures may be practised separately .The programme may be summarized as consisting of:

Corpse Posture (*Savasana*), for relaxation
Spinal Rock, a warm-up exercise
Shoulderstand Posture (*Sarvangasana*)
Incline-board or tilt-chair
Plough Posture (*Halasana*)
Fish Posture (*Matsyasana*)
Back-stretching Posture (*Paschimottanasana*)
Cobra Posture (*Bhujangasana*)
Bow Posture (*Dhanurasana*)
Corpse Posture (*Savasana*)

Readers should go on to plan individual and carefully graduated programmes from the 418 postures described in *Yoga Postures*, where they are divided into Warm-ups, and Groups A and B. The two groups are based on the difficulty of the postures, and each of the three sections is subdivided into standing postures, sitting and kneeling postures, supine postures, prone postures, inverted postures, and muscular locks. The advanced Group B has an additional section on balancing postures. Each of the three sections – Warm-ups, Group A and Group B – concludes with instructions on how

to plan programmes to suit individual needs. Many variations on
the main traditional poses are given and an additional section
summarizes the therapeutic powers claimed for the *asanas*.

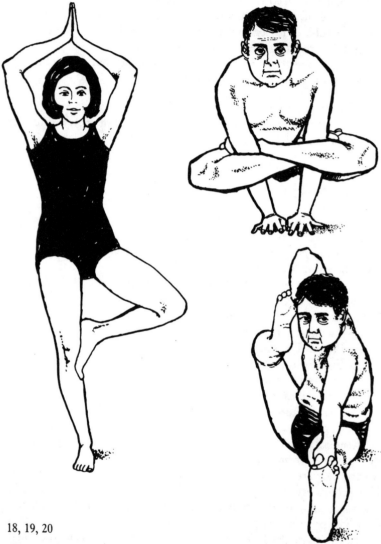

18, 19, 20

Three advanced poses, whose performance is described in Yoga of
Posture: Tree Posture: Vrkasana; Cock Posture: Kukutasana; Shooting
Bow Posture: Akaran Dhanurasana.

IV Yogic Hygiene

THE SIX CLEANSING ACTS

If any reader needs convincing that the men who devised the system of bodily, mental, and spiritual perfecting that is Yoga brought a thoroughness to their experiments that resulted in unique, strange, but effective practices, let him look at the six main cleansing duties (*kriyas*) or acts (*shatkarmas*) of the Hatha Yogins. Even if he does not wish to practise them all – at least not in their traditional form – he will have to admit that here is personal hygiene carried to astounding lengths and displaying a remarkable knowledge of the human body.

A warning must be given. Only a few Westerners perform the more severe of these purifications in their traditional form, and then always under the personal supervision of a teacher. But modern adaptations are possible in several cases, and these readers may wish to try. Certainly there is no need to miss *Nauli* and *Kapalabhati*, the last two of the six hygienic duties. The former, with its preliminary muscle control of *Uddiyana Bandha*, has a chapter to itself, and *Kapalabhati* is included in the chapter on Yogic Breath Control (*Pranayama*).

The six hygienic duties (*kriyas*), as given by the *Hatha Yoga Pradipika*, are *Dhauti*, *Basti* (or *Vasti*), *Neti*, *Trataka*, *Nauli*, and *Kapalabhati*. The *Gheranda Samhita* substitutes *Lauliki* for *Nauli*. The duties are used as preparatory cleansing to ensure the full benefits of the breathing exercises (*pranayama*) and to improve health by removing impurities, phlegm, and excess fat. The breathing exercises have themselves a purificatory role, and *Kapalabhati* is itself a respiratory exercise. The six *kriyas* cleanse the respiratory, digestive, eliminatory, and nervous systems. To quote Sir Paul Dukes (20): 'In the last analysis physical health depends on the efficient working of the following four processes: elimination, alimentation, respiration, and relaxation. These are referred to in esoteric schools as the Sacred Physical Arts.' Alimentation (nourishment), respiration, and relaxation are in this book given their own chapters. We will be mainly concerned in this chapter with cleansing by elimination of toxic material.

DHAUTI (WASHING)

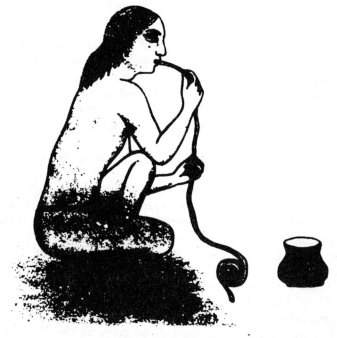

21

Dhauti (Washing)

A long strip of cloth – surgical gauze can be used – three to four inches wide, is soaked in warm water or milk. It is then swallowed slowly and carefully and allowed to rest in the stomach for ten to fifteen minutes before being pulled out slowly. If you leave the strip of cloth in the stomach longer than twenty minutes it begins to pass through the body. Dr Bernard swallowed the whole strip, and had to retrieve it with an emetic of salt and water. A tendency to retch during first attempts passes with practice. At first only two or three feet should be swallowed; this may increase gradually to fifteen feet or more as the lining of the throat becomes accustomed to the practice.

In *Dhauti* (which means 'to wash') the swallowed cloth soaks up phlegm, bile, and other impurities in the stomach. The process is taught at Yoga therapy centres in India, and is said to cure many diseases. The *Hatha Yoga Pradipika* says (75): 'There is no doubt that cough, asthma, enlargement of the spleen, leprosy, and twenty kinds of diseases born of phlegm disappear by the practice of Dhauti Karma.'

An alternative, with somewhat similar benefits, is to drink several glasses of warm water in which a teaspoonful of salt has been dissolved, until vomiting empties the stomach. This is called *Vamana Dhauti*. Some Yogins develop the ability to vomit at will and cleanse the stomach. Houdini, the famous escapologist, taught himself this art, regurgitating a key that enabled him to unlock a trunk inside which he seemed trapped.

The *Gheranda Samhita* describes four kinds of *Dhauti*: *Antardhauti* or internal washing (itself divided into four parts); *Dantadhauti* or cleaning the teeth; *Hrd-dhauti* or cleaning the chest or throat; and *Mula-sodhana* or cleaning the rectum.

Antar-dhauti (Internal Washing)
The four parts of *Antar-dhauti* are *Vatasara* or air purification, *Varisara* or water purification, *Vahnisara* or fire purification, and *Bahiskrta* or cleansing the intestines.

Air Purification (*Vatasara*): contracting the mouth into the shape of a crow's beak, draw in air slowly, until the stomach feels comfortably full. Move the air in the stomach for a short time, and then release it slowly from the rectum. The *Gheranda Samhita* says (87): 'The *Vatsara* is a very secret process, it causes the purification of the body, it destroys all diseases and increases the gastric fire.'

Water Purification (*Varisara*): take a mouthful of water, and then drink it slowly. Move the water in the stomach; then take it downwards, and release it through the rectum. The *Gheranda Samhita* says (87): 'This process should be kept secret. It purifies the body. And by practising it with care, one gets a luminous or shining body.

The *Varisara* is the highest *Dhauti*. He who practises it with ease, purifies his filthy body and turns it into a shining one.'

Fire Purification (*Vahnisara*): 'Press the navel knot or intestines back towards the spine for one hundred times.' In Yogic physiology the region behind the navel is a place of fire or heat, which is kindled by this instroke. A beginner should commence with five instrokes to one exhalation, and increase gradually over several weeks until he is performing ten. Digestion is aided and the abdominal viscera are massaged. The *Gheranda Samhita* says (87): 'This is *Agnisara* or fire process. This gives success in the practice of Yoga, it cures all the diseases of the stomach [gastric juice] and increases the internal fire. This form of *Dhauti* should be kept very secret, and it is hardly to be attained even by the gods. By this *Dhauti* alone one gets a luminous body.' (*See also* the chapter on Abdominal Retraction.)

Intestinal Purification (*Bahiskrta*): here again we are brought up with a jolt at the lengths to which Yogins go to cleanse the body internally. Readers should *not* attempt this hygienic practice, which has two parts. First, the stomach is filled with air, drawn in by the crow's beak method described for Air Purification. The air is held in the stomach for an hour and a half, and then moved down to the intestines. The second part brings the jolt. Standing in water up to the navel, the Yogin draws out the long intestine (*saktinadi*) and washes it with both hands – the *Gheranda Samhita* says (87): 'wash it with care, and then draw it in again into the abdomen. This process should be kept secret. It is not easily to be attained even by the gods. Simply by this *Dhauti* one gets *Deva-deha* [godlike body.]'

Danta-dhauti (Cleaning the Teeth)
This includes cleaning the gums, the tongue, the ears, and the frontal sinuses.

Teeth Cleansing (*Danta-mula-dhauti*). the teeth and gums are rubbed every morning with catechu plant powder or pure earth.

Tongue Cleansing (*Jihva-sodhana*): the *Gheranda Samhita* says (87):
Join together the three fingers known as the index, the middle and the ring finger, put them into the throat, and rub well and clean the root of the tongue, and by washing it again throw out the phlegm. Having

thus washed it rub it with butter, and milk it again and again; then by holding the tip of the tongue with an iron instrument pull it out slowly and slowly. By so doing, the tongue becomes elongated.

The text says earlier: 'The elongation of the tongue destroys old age, death and disease.' Lengthening the tongue also has a role in some esoteric practices in which the passing of air through the nostrils is blocked by curling the tongue back in the mouth.

Ear Cleansing (*Karna-dhauti*): the text (87) is concise: 'Clean the two holes of the ears by the index and the ring fingers. By practising it daily, the mystical sounds are heard.'

Cleansing the Frontal Sinuses (*Kapalarandhra-dhauti*): the *Gheranda Samhita* directs (87):
Rub with the thumb of the right hand the depression in the forehead near the bridge of the nose. By the practice of this Yoga, diseases arising from derangements of phlegmatic humours are cured. The vessels become purified and clairvoyance is induced. This should be practised daily after awakening from sleep, after meals, and in the evening.

Hrd-dhauti (Cleansing the Chest or Throat)
Three methods are employed:

With a Stalk (*Danda-dhauti*): a stalk of plantain, turmeric or cane is slowly pushed into the gullet and then drawn out slowly. Thereby, says the *Gheranda Samhita* (87): 'phlegm, bile and other impurities are expelled out of the mouth.' The practice is also considered good for the heart.

With Water (*Vamana-dhauti*): the *Gheranda Samhita* directs (87): 'After meal, let the wise practitioner drink water full up to the throat, then looking for a short while upwards, let him vomit it out again. By daily practising this Yoga, disorders of the phlegm and bile are cured.' This is an example of the ambiguity of much instruction in the old texts. Professor Wood (91) interprets this as 'cleansing by gargling,' but the word 'vomit' would seem to indicate that water is filled 'up to the throat' from the stomach upwards, and this is indeed the way Theos Bernard was taught – an alternative to swallowing surgical gauze.

With a Strip of Cloth (*Vaso-dhauti*): this is the first method described under *Dhauti*.

Mula-sodhana (Cleansing the Rectum)
The rectum is cleaned internally with water, 'over and over again', using the middle finger of one hand or a stalk of turmeric (yellow sandal).

BASTI OR VASTI (COLONIC IRRIGATION)

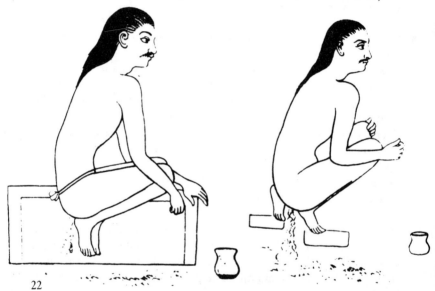

22

Basti (Colonic Irrigation)

The *Gheranda Samhita* gives two kinds of *Vasti*: *Jala-Vasti* (Water *Vasti*) and *Suska Vasti* (Dry *Vasti*). The first is performed squatting on the heels in water up to the navel and contracting and dilating the sphincters of the anus, letting water into the colon, holding it there for a time and churning it about, and then releasing it by opening the anal sphincters. A vacuum in the colon is created by performing an Abdominal Retraction (*Uddiyana Bandha*) on squatting, and the water is churned about by means of Recti Isolation (*Nauli*). These two abdominal controls are given a chapter to themselves. A greased enema nozzle may be inserted by persons who have not yet mastered the control of the sphincters. Yogins hold their natural method of colonic cleansing to be superior to the use of the modern enema. Western writers on Yoga are divided as to whether or not use of natural colonic irrigation or an enema is desirable. Some take the view that the practices of Yoga ensure regular bowel evacuation and that nothing more need be done. The present writer has so far belonged to this group, those 'playing safe', though he is conscious that he (and his readers) may be missing out on a valuable cleansing practice no more 'unnatural' than brushing the teeth. Sir Paul Dukes, a strong advocate of the Yogic enema, gives detailed instructions for its use in his book *The Yoga of Health, Youth, and Joy* (20). The *Gheranda Samhita* says (87): 'The body becomes free from all diseases and becomes as beautiful as the god Cupid.'

In Dry *Basti* or *Vasti* you begin by adopting the Back-stretching Posture (*Paschimottanasana*). Sit on the floor with both legs fully extended together, locked at the knees. Then lean slowly forward from the waist and lower the head as far as you can towards the knees (experts bring the face against the knees), at the same time reaching forward to grasp either the ankles or the feet. Now press the intestines down and squeeze tightly the muscles of the anus. This is called *Asvini* or Horse *Mudra*, as it imitates the staling of a horse. The *Gheranda Samhita* says (87): 'By this practice of Yoga, constipation never occurs, and it increases gastric fire and cures flatulence.'

BLADDER IRRIGATION

This is more difficult than colonic irrigation by muscle control. Water is drawn up the urethra to cleanse the bladder. Some Hatha Yogins can manage it.

NETI (NASAL CLEANSING)

This is a practice for clearing the nostrils and the head sinuses. There are two techniques: one using a catheter and the other using water.

A thin catheter, lubricated with antiseptic jelly, should be passed up one nostril until the end appears in the throat, when it is gripped

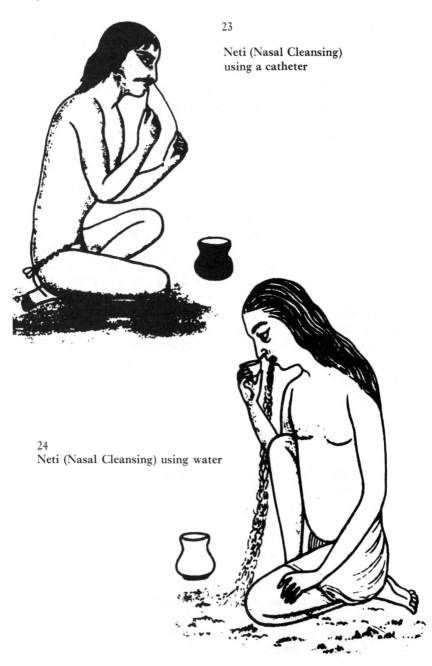

23

Neti (Nasal Cleansing)
using a catheter

24
Neti (Nasal Cleansing) using water

between the thumb and forefinger of one hand and drawn out through the mouth. With one end protruding from the mouth and the other from the nostril, gently and slowly draw the catheter to and fro a few times before finally pulling its full length out of the mouth. The traditional method is to use a soft cord, but a catheter is the modern, and safer, device. Clear first one nostril, and then the other.

Many readers will prefer the alternative method, using water, though an uncomfortable sensation in the nostrils has to be overcome by repeated practice. Lukewarm water (previously boiled), to which a teaspoonful of salt has been added, is sniffed from a cup, a saucer, or the cupped hand up both nostrils and then expelled from the mouth. This is called *Vyut-krama*. You can also fill the mouth with water and expel it through the nostrils. This is called *Sit-krama*. A nasal douche may be found more comfortable for cleansing the nostrils.

The *Gheranda Samhita*, with characteristic exaggeration, says (87), 'by this practice of Yoga one becomes like the god Cupid. Old age never comes to him and decrepitude never disfigures him. The body becomes healthy, elastic, and disorders due to phlegm are destroyed.' The practice also has a reputation for improving the vision and bringing a concomitant *claritas* to consciousness.

TRATAKA (CLEANSING VISION)

In this practice an object is gazed at without blinking until the eyes begin to water. Do not stare – *look*. This means looking *through* the eyes, rather than staring *from* them. This exercise is also found in the Yoga of Meditation – a candle flame or a flower is a favoured focus of attention. The practitioner is instructed to sit calmly with the back straight for this concentration, which steadies the mind as well as the body and the gaze.

An occult tradition says that *Trataka* induces powers of clairvoyance, which is perhaps why an old text says the practice 'should be kept secret carefully, like a box of jewellery.'

Stop *Trataka* immediately the eyes begin to water. Bathe them with cold water, and then move them about in the Clock Exercise. You imagine a large clock face about three feet in front of the face and, without moving the head, look up at twelve o'clock, down to

six o'clock, up to one o'clock, diagonally down to seven o'clock, up
to two o'clock and across to eight o'clock, and so on round the clock
face. Repeat in an anti-clockwise direction.

NAULI (RECTI ISOLATION)

For this exercise, see the separate chapter devoted to it.

LAULIKI (ABDOMINAL ROLLING)

The *Gheranda Samhita* (87) substitutes *Lauliki* for *Nauli*. They are
on similar lines, though *Lauliki* can be used by students who have
not yet mastered *Nauli*. 'With great force move the stomach and
intestines from one side to the other. This is called Lauliki-Yoga.
This destroys all diseases and increases the bodily fire.'
    This is a general rolling of the abdomen, instead of isolation of
the vertical recti muscles (as in *Nauli*). *Nauli* is superior, and one
should endeavour to master it, first attaining perfect performance of
the preliminary Abdominal Retraction (*Uddiyana Bandha*).

KAPALABHATI (CLEANSING BREATH)

For a description of this exercise, see the chapter on Yogic breath
control (*pranayama*).

HYGIENIC ACHIEVEMENT

Some Westerners find some of the practices described above
grotesque and distasteful, perhaps associating them with the self-
mortification of Indian fakirs and so-called 'holy men' – beds of
nails, withered limbs, and so on. The comparison, if made, is totally
unjust. The purification processes described show a mastery of the
body and a regard for cleanliness that should make the average
occidental shamefaced. However, readers are free to ignore or use
any of the *kriyas*. But whatever the decision, it would be unfair not
to recognize them as a remarkable hygienic achievement.

In conclusion, it should be noted that *all* the practices of Hatha Yoga are purificatory. Yogic postures, breath controls, and diet all remove impurities from the body and cleanse the bloodstream; and the practice of meditation is a mental hygiene, making consciousness more lucid and, in Blake's phrase, 'cleansing the doors of perception.'

V Abdominal Retraction and Recti Isolation

ABDOMINAL RETRACTION (*UDDIYANA BANDHA*)

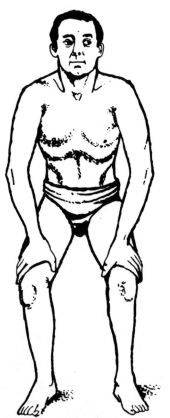

Abdominal Retraction: Uddiyana Bandha

'*Uddiyana Bandha* is a blessing to mankind; it brings health, strength and long life to those who practise it. For abdominal exercises nothing can compete with *Uddiyana* and *Nauli*. They stand unique, unrivalled and unprecedented, amongst all systems of physical exercises in the East and West.' So wrote Swami Sivananda, whose *ashram* is in the foothills of the Himalayas.

In *Uddiyana* the abdominal wall is retracted on empty lungs, creating a deep hollow. 'Make the abdomen look quite hollow just like a tank,' says the *Gheranda Samhita*. After mastering this muscle control, the two recti muscles can be isolated in the centre of the abdomen (*Nauli*). An even more advanced control is the isolation of the left rectus and the right rectus alternately, creating a wave-like motion across the abdomen from side to side.

The two muscle controls are treated in the classic texts as purifactory practices, but here we utilize them as matchless exercises for abdominal health.

Bandha means 'binding', and *Uddiyana* comes from the Sanskrit roots *ut* and *di*, and means 'to fly upwards'. *Prana* or life-force is said to fly upwards via the *sushuma nadi* or main channel of the subtle body. 'To fly' implies speed, but in this esoteric tradition it usually takes several hours of intense concentration and breath and muscle control to take the internal energies upwards to the crown of the head.

To the onlooker, the spectacle of this muscle control is either impressive or revolting. Women are more likely to show disapproval than men, who usually rush home to practice before a mirror – though Arthur Koestler, in *The Yogi and the Commissar*, described it as 'fascinating and faintly nauseating.' The visual impression is, however, of no great importance – what *is* important is the health value of the control.

Technique
   i. It is found that control is facilitated in early practice by standing with the legs a little apart and slightly bent at the knee, the kneecaps directly above the toes – the skiing position. *The palm of the right hand is placed on top of the right thigh and the palm of the left hand on top of the left thigh, the fingers spread a little and pointing inwards. The arms are fully stretched, the trunk leans forward slightly from the waist, and the back is rounded a little. Later you should be able to perform* Uddiyana *and* Nauli *in other standing and sitting*

positions. The Lotus Posture and other sitting postures are often used by Yogins for these two muscle controls.

ii. *Empty the lungs thoroughly. Success depends on this. The lungs are kept empty throughout the control.* In pranayama *the emptying is usually performed slowly and smoothly through the nostrils, but here you should empty the lungs as fast as possible through both nostrils and mouth. If you take too long over this stage you will have to fight an urge to take an inbreath, which disturbs performance of the control.*

iii. *Relax the abdominal wall, keeping the lungs emptied of air. Now expand the thoracic cage as though to make a thoracic inspiration – but actually only go through the motions of expanding the ribs, without taking in air. A slight lift of the thoracic cage is usually found helpful.*

iv. *The diaphragm will now move up into the thoracic cavity and the stomach will travel inwards, as though being pulled by a wire attached to the base of the backbone. Hold the retraction for a few seconds, and then release the abdominal wall smoothly. If you let it spring back with a jerk, the inrush of air will be explosive, which is faulty Yoga practice.*

What happens is that emptying the lungs and expanding the thorax causes the abdomen to move back to fill the vacuum created. This should be effortless. A deep hollow appears, in which both fists could be placed. Fat stomachs make *Uddiyana* and *Nauli* difficult, and women, with their extra fat, find these controls, especially *Nauli*, more difficult than men. The Abdominal Retraction is demonstrated by Lady Dukes (20). In classic performance, when the abdomen is fully retracted, the *oblique* muscles stand out like cords. Those of the Yogin observed by Arthur Koestler did. An exceptionally lean abdomen is needed to display this crowning touch, and few book illustrations show it. It is Dr Theos Bernard, an American, who depicts it best in Plate xxxiii of his *Hatha Yoga*. He also shows cleanly-executed central isolation of the recti, and the left rectus and the right rectus separately. Some Indian experts, though remarkably supple, show a surprisingly large amount of waistline flab – though it must be pointed out that the hard 'washboard' effect cultivated by Western weight-training body-builders is neither aimed at nor thought desirable in India.

Developing Skill

Yoga's Abdominal Retraction is unique: no other exercise comes near to matching it for squeezing and kneading the viscera – intestines, spleen, pancreas, liver, kidneys, transverse colon – or for toning the supporting muscular 'corset'.

The exercise should be performed on an empty stomach. This means that immediately after rising in the morning is the best time for practice. Two methods should be employed. The first is to hold the retraction for five seconds, and then release the abdomen and breathe normally for a few seconds. Exhale again and repeat the retraction. Perform five times to make up a cycle. The second method is to perform five fast retractions and releases on one emptying of the lungs. This counts as one cycle. Perform as smoothly as possible, taking no air into the lungs. During the first month perform three cycles, during the second month four cycles, and during the third month and thereafter five cycles. This applies to both methods. Later you may wish to include an extra session of practice daily, and to add Recti Isolation.

Agnisari Dhauti
This means literally 'purification through fire' – the digestive fire, that is. It is really the first of the two methods of practice described above, but prolonged. It is only recommended for advanced practitioners. A series of retractions is performed on one exhalation of air. As soon as the maximum hollowing has been achieved, the abdominal wall is released, and immediately drawn back again. The viscera are powerfully massaged and the digestive fires are fanned. Under *ashram* conditions, Yogins may perform as many as 1,500 retractions in one day, but readers should never exceed a number that feels comfortable and beneficial. (*See also* Fire Purification (*Vahnisara*) in the chapter on Yoga Hygiene.)

RECTI ISOLATION (*NAULI*)

The recti abdominis are the straight muscles of the abdomen, lying side by side in vertical strips down the centre of the abdomen from chest bone to pubic bone. The ability to isolate them consciously is another of Yoga's remarkable discoveries about the human body. Success in *Nauli* will not come until you have mastered *Uddiyana* to the extent that a very deep hollow is effortlessly created. Keeping the lungs empty of air, you then isolate the recti by pushing them forward, as though they have stepped forward from a deep cave to

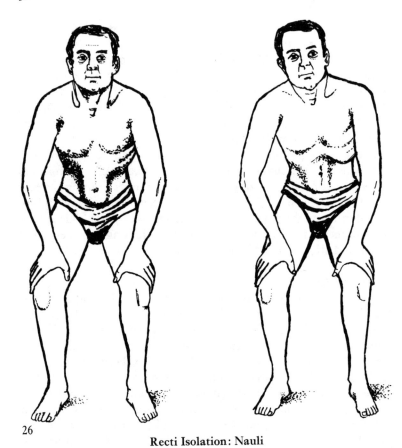

26

Recti Isolation: Nauli

stand motionless at its entrance. Practising before a mirror helps in the early stages, and slight pressure downwards of the palms of the hands is another aid. Later, both these aids can be dropped.

As soon as you are proficient in *Nauli*, add its practice to that of *Uddiyana Bandha*, performing it in the two ways indicated for *Uddiyana* and with the same number of repetitions.

Lateral Abdominal Rolling
This is the acme of Yogic control of the abdominal muscles. The right rectus is isolated by itself; then the left rectus isolated; then right; then left; and so on in a continuous wave-like motion that crosses the abdomen from right to left and from left to right. Good

form is essential; speed can be worked up gradually. The number of successive 'waves' will depend on how long you can comfortably suspend breathing. Always stay within the borders of comfort. Recti rolling gives the abdominal muscles and viscera the maximum churning, squeezing, and kneading.

BENEFITS

No exercises superior to these have been devised for what F. A. Hornibrook called 'culture of the abdomen'. Even if you do not progress to Recti Isolation or Lateral Abdominal Rolling, all the benefits described are obtained to some extent by retracting the abdomen (*Uddiyana Bandha*).

In Kundalini Yoga these controls are used to awaken the body's dormant electro-magnetic energies. On a practical level, they firm, tone, and trim the abdomen; massage the viscera; clear congestion caused by sedentary habits and the upright stance; correct constipation; improve digestion; and stimulate the liver, pancreas, kidneys, spleen, and adrenal glands. They are linked with sexual vigour and the overcoming of sexual disabilities. The diaphragm is encouraged to move, to become more mobile, and thus to perform better the up-and-down piston-like movement that operates deep and healthful breathing. The important solar plexus region is stimulated. Elasticity of the lungs is improved, and the heart is said to receive a gentle massage obtainable in no other way. The abdominal muscles and internal organs receive a kneading and squeezing superior to what could be got from the hands of an expert masseur. The viscera are lifted and squeezed against the spine. Repeated uplift prevents prolapse. Metabolism, circulation, and digestion are stimulated.

The controls are unrivalled as aids to natural and regular bowel action. Constipation is corrected long-term, not momentarily treated as by taking a laxative. An Indian doctor, Vasant G. Rele, who made a study of the physiological effects of Hatha Yoga practices, wrote (68):

Excessive activity of the sympathetic nervous system inhibits peristaltic activity of the intestines and produces constipation. On the other hand, an excessive activity of the parasympathetic increases the movements of the intestines, and produces looseness of the bowels. . . . By the practice of *Uddiyana Bandha* the excessive activity of the sympathetic

nervous system is controlled without exciting the parasympathetic,
overstimulation of which would create a vicious circle. . . . The sudden
retraction of the relaxed abdominal muscles, particularly the two recti
(straight front muscles of the abdomen), against the spine after their
preliminary contraction in the full expiratory effort in the practice of
Uddiyana Bandha, drags the intestines upwards and downwards to
their utmost limit. This stretches with them the sympathetic fibres
curbing any tendency towards overactivity of the solar plexus – the
brain of the sympathetic nervous system – without the stimulation of
the parasympethetic.

Abdominal Retraction (*Uddiyana Bandha*) and Recti Isolation
(*Nauli*), in common with other forms of Yoga practice, are thus seen
to have a beneficial influence on the nervous system and, through it,
the functioning of the whole psycho-physical organism.

THE BREATH OF LIFE

Many physiological processes are essential to human life: the
functioning of the heart, the regulation of the temperature, and so
on. All must work together for us to survive. But one physiological
function seems to us most intimately connected with life – *breathing*.
'Breath is life,' the Yogins say. And few treatises on *pranayama*
omit to mention that we can survive for weeks without food, and
for days without water, but that our survival without air has to be
measured in seconds.

The dominion of breath over the senses is expressed in many old
Sanskrit texts, and perhaps most poetically in the *Brihadaranyaka
Upanishad* (114):

The senses, when quarrelling together as to who was the best, went to
Brahman and said: 'Who is the richest of us?' He replied: 'He by
whose departure the body seems worst, he is the richest.'

The tongue [speech] departed, and having been absent for a year,
it came back and said: 'How have you been able to live without me?'
They replied: 'Like unto people, not speaking with the tongue, but
breathing with breath, seeing with the eye, hearing with the ear,
knowing with the mind, generating with seed. Thus we have lived.'
Then speech entered in.

The eye [sight] departed, and having been absent for a year, it
came back and said: 'How have you been able to live without me?'
They replied: 'Like blind people not seeing with the eye, but breathing

with the breath, speaking with the tongue, hearing with the ear, knowing with the mind, generating with seed. Thus we have lived.' Then the eye entered in.

The ear [hearing] departed, and having been absent for a year, it came back and said: 'How have you been able to live without me?' They replied: 'Like deaf people, not hearing with the ear, but breathing with the breath, speaking with the tongue, seeing with the eye, knowing with the mind, generating with seed. Thus we have lived.' Then the ear entered in.

The mind departed, and having been absent for a year, it came back and said: 'How have you been able to live without me?' They replied: 'Like fools, not knowing with the mind, but breathing with the breath, seeing with the eye, hearing with the ear, generating with seed. Thus we have lived.' Then the mind entered in.

The seed departed, and having been absent for a year, it came back and said: 'How have you been able to live without me?' They replied: 'Like impotent people, not generating with seed, but breathing with the breath, seeing with the eye, hearing with the ear, knowing with the mind. Thus we have lived.' Then the seed entered in.

The [vital] breath, when on the point of departure, tore up these senses, as a great, excellent horse of the Sindhu country might tear up the pegs to which he is tethered. They said to him: 'Sir, do not depart. We shall not be able to live without thee.'

PRANAYAMA DEFINED

Pranayama, the Yogic science of breath control, is at the very heart of Hatha Yoga practice. Basically, Hatha Yoga is mastery of body and of breath. Sir Paul Dukes, who studied and taught Yoga in India, says (20) that purification is the keynote of Hatha Yoga, and the foremost practice of purification is *pranayama*. For this reason, breath control is more important than the *asanas* or postures, though ideally both should be an integral part of the Hatha Yoga system. Breathing exercises are considered essential for the preliminary purification whereby the cells and nerve channels are cleansed and made ready for advanced control of subtle inner energies.

The Sanskrit word *hatha* has associations with breathing. In Yogic tradition the flow of breath through the right nostril is controlled by the sun, and that through the left nostril by the moon.

The Sanskrit *ha* means 'sun' and *tha* means 'moon'. The air that travels through the right nostril (*pingala*) is positive ('sun breath') and that which travels through the left nostril (*ida*) is negative ('moon breath'). The word *yoga* means 'union'. Hatha Yoga thus unifies the positive and negative, male and female, sun and moon universal principles within the human organism. This balancing of energy currents is subjectively experienced as a state of inner poise and equilibrium. Controlled breathing (*pranayama*) is the key practice for attaining this desirable physiological and psychical state.

In the eight 'limbs' (*angas*) of classical Yoga as mapped out by Patanjali, breath control comes after bodily poses (*asanas*), and before withdrawal of the senses from external objects (*pratyahara*), the first step in turning the attention inwards for concentration (*dharana*) and its extension as contemplation (*dhyana*), leading to the superconscious experience of *samadhi*.

Yogic breath control operates at several levels, from the exoteric boosting of vitality and health to esoteric approaches to mystical states of consciousness. A multiplicity of benefits accrue from raising the level of general health and from having rich reserves of energy. The mind benefits from the calming and toning of the nervous system, and the tone and texture of consciousness itself is influenced by the rate and rhythm of respiration and by pausing between inhalation and exhalation and between exhalation and inhalation. *Pranayama* prepares the mind for the meditative practices of Raja Yoga, and breathing may itself become the object of concentration and contemplation. Breathing meditation is found in the practices of Hindu, Taoist, Buddhist, Zen, and Sufist mysticism.

The term *pranayama* is made up of two parts. One meaning of *prana* is 'breath'. *Yama* belongs to the ethical foundation of Yoga practice: it means 'restraint' or 'control'. *Pranayama* is therefore in one sense 'breath control'. The breath flow into and out of the lungs is regulated, and made smooth and slow in most exercises. Sometimes first one nostril is used while the other is closed, and then the roles of the nostrils are reversed. Breathing is suspended at the end of each inhalation or exhalation. For normal purposes this should only be for a few seconds – holding the breath to the point of discomfort or strain could be damaging to health, whereas controlled breathing well within capacity enhances health. Readers should not anticipate essaying any remarkable feats in this direction.

Yama has another related meaning, given by Archie Bahm (5) as: 'persisting disposition or enduring nature or tendency to retain strength,' to which definition he adds a rider in keeping with our practical approach: 'to interpret *yama* as sustained relaxation, and *pranayama* as a way of sustaining unanxious living through healthy breathing habits, would not be inappropriate.' Yogic breathing relaxes body and mind. But this is a peripheral definition.

We have given one definition of *prana* – 'breath'. *Prana* has also wider connotations, described below.

PRANA

Translating *prana* as 'life breath' rather than 'breath' goes some way towards indicating its broader dimension. *Prana* is the power within breath and 'the vital force in every being'. As cosmic energy, it pervades everything. It is a vital substance not yet covered by scientific classification, though it should be noted that the modern physicists' discovery that 'all is energy' recalls statements on the origins of the universe and its evolution made by Yogic philosophers many centuries ago. *Prana* is the life-force within and about us. It operates in the working of our respiration, circulation, digestion, and other body processes, and is at the same time the universal life-force in which we share. An ocean of energy is at our disposal and through Yoga we can learn how to tap it.

Vivekananda, in his *Raja Yoga*, expressed this concept with characteristic eloquence:

In an ocean there are huge waves, then smaller waves, and still smaller, down to little bubbles; but back of all these is an infinite ocean. The bubble is connected with the infinite ocean at one end, and the huge wave at the other end. So, one may be a gigantic man, and another a little bubble, but each is connected with that infinite ocean of energy which is the common birthright of every animal that exists. Wherever there is life, the storehouse of that infinite energy is behind it.

Air is strongly charged with *prana*, and it is potently present in sunlight and in the foods we eat, especially those that are sun-ripened. Air being the most vital of all foods, improved breathing methods mean a richer supply of *prana*, that is, of life itself. Disease is unlikely to gain a hold in a body whose tissues and organs are charged with *prana*.

Apart from the *prana* absorbed from air and food, Hatha Yogins say that there are concentrations of *prana* stored within the body. These, coiled and latent, are sources of physiological and psychic power, which *pranayama* helps activate. This comes within the practice of Kundalini Yoga, also called Laya Yoga, which will be discussed in a later section.

In Yogic breathing, *prana* – both as breath and as vital cosmic force – is gathered and utilized to physiological, mental, and spiritual advantage. The spiritual side is only a peripheral concern of Yoga of Vitality, but one is reminded of it by Tennyson's words, 'Closer is He than breathing, and nearer than hands and feet.' The poet was referring to the personal God of Christianity, but for the pure Yoga of the *upanishads* one must substitute *Brahman*, the impersonal Absolute, in pure consciousness the ground of Being.

In breathing we make our most intimate contact with the cosmic life force, which is why the Yogins consider breath control to be of primary importance, and why breath is given dominion over the senses and other physiological processes in Yoga's classic texts and in the sublime *upanishads*.

FAULTY BREATHING

Only a minority of adults in civilized countries breathe with full efficiency and for maximum healthful effect. Young children, unless they have some bodily defect, breathe more effectively than adults, but once they are subjected to social pressures and tensions they develop the faulty respiratory habits of their parents, principally shallow high-chest breathing.

If great numbers of people have lost the technique of using their respiratory muscles and lungs with adequate elasticity, the result can only be destructive to health. The bloodstream is not being fully purified and oxygenated, nor is food being adequately burned in the body to provide energy. It also goes a long way to explaining the prevalence of fatigue, headaches, and neurasthenia in civilized life.

Breathing deeply, for great numbers of people, has to be re-learned, and shallow upper-chest inhalation replaced by diaphragmatic and abdominal breathing, of the kind visible in sleeping infants.

To understand the physiological basis of what is involved in breathing deeply and healthfully, it is helpful to acquire knowledge of the basic facts of the anatomy and physiology of respiration. Readers wishing to extend their knowledge beyond the summary given here can find suitable textbooks on anatomy and physiology in bookshops and libraries.

MAN'S NEED FOR OXYGEN

Scientists believe that several hundred million years ago all living organisms on our planet lived in the sea. Later the first amphibian managed to live in both water and air. Even now only fifteen per cent of living organisms exist on land and breathe the earth's oxygen-charged atmosphere. For man's living on dry land he has to thank his hard-working lungs, which take in oxygen, process it, and transfer it to the blood.

The earth's atmosphere contains twenty-one per cent oxygen. On it consciousness itself depends: if the oxygen level in the atmosphere surrounding us falls, we rapidly become unconscious.

Our billions of body cells need to breathe; more exactly, they need to receive oxygen and to return carbon dioxide, the waste product of metabolic activities within the cells. The lungs pass oxygen from the air we breathe into the blood, which is carried to the cells. The circulating bloodstream also carries the waste gases, and the lungs expel carbon dioxide on our outgoing breaths.

Oxygen could be described as our most essential food. It is essential for the metabolic processes on which our vitality depends. Burning up food produces energy in much the same way as burning up petrol in the engine of an automobile provides power. A large and constant supply of oxygen is needed for the combustion of food products (oxidation). The amount we absorb through the skin is insufficient for our needs, so we must depend on the efficient functioning of our respiratory muscles and organs.

THE RESPIRATORY TRACT

The main components of the respiratory tract are the nostrils, the pharynx, the larynx, the trachea (windpipe), the bronchi, and the lungs.

Yogic (and healthy) breathing uses the nose and not the mouth. The nasal passages are lined with fine hairs, which act as filters and trap dust and bacteria, and with mucous membrane, which warms and moistens the incoming air. The nose is divided by the septum into two narrow passages. In some *pranayama* exercises alternate nostrils are used: this tends to produce a relaxing effect.

Inhaled air, having been drawn up the nostrils, passes into the pharynx, the cavity behind and communicating with the nose, mouth, and larynx. The vocal cords normally are not vibrated in *pranayama* (though they are in Mantra Yoga, which is based on vocalizing), but there are one or two Yogic breathing exercises in which the glottis, which modulates the voice, is half-closed.

The windpipe or trachea is about four and a half inches in length and one inch in diameter. The word 'trachea' derives from the Greek *trakhus*, meaning 'rough'. The roughness, which can be felt in the throat with the fingertips, is caused by alternate rings of cartilage and fibrous tissue.

The windpipe enters the thoracic cavity at the neck and divides into the right bronchus and the left bronchus, which supply air to the right and left lungs respectively. Trachea and bronchi are hollow tubes which stay open due to the cartilaginous rings in their walls. The unpleasant bronchitis is an infection of the bronchi. From each bronchus radiate smaller branches, which ramify into a bronchial tree composed of fine bronchioles, ending in clusters of air-filled sacs called alveoli, which contain blood vessels. There are about 750 million air sacs or alveoli in the lungs, an indication of their tiny size.

The lungs are not of equal size: the right lung is slightly the larger of the two and has three lobes to the left lung's two. If a diseased lobe is removed, the others carry the extra work. Adult lungs weigh from two to two and a half pounds, and if the lining could be spread out flat it would cover about a hundred square yards of ground. Healthy lungs that have enjoyed nothing but fresh air are pink; those of heavy smokers are purple-black.

The mucous membrane lining the respiratory tract has goblet cells and hair-like cilia. The mucus keeps the windpipe and bronchi moist. The cilia, moving always in one direction, trap particles of dirt and sweep them up towards the mouth. If the cilia are faced with too much work, a spasm of coughing is triggered, in the same way that too much dust or dirt in the nostrils sets off a sneeze.

Each lung is enveloped by a double layer of smooth membrane, which prevents any friction that might arise from movements of the lungs against the rib-cage. The inner layer of this protective membrane is called the visceral pleura and the outer layer the parietal pleura. Pleurisy is inflammation of the pleura, and pneumonia is inflammation of the lungs.

THE THORACIC CAGE

The bony thoracic cage, which houses the heart and lungs, is of intricate construction and quite narrow at its apex, though the shoulders to each side give an impression to the contrary. At the front is the breastbone or sternum; at the back are the twelve thoracic vertebrae of the spinal column; on each flank are the ribs – twelve pairs, whose interstices are filled by the intercostal muscles, nerves, and blood vessels. The top seven pairs are known as the true ribs; the eighth, ninth, and tenth pairs as false ribs, joining up with the ribs above and in the breastbone; and the two pairs of short bottom ribs which join into the abdomen are called floating ribs.

It is the expansion of the ribs that initiates the act of breathing.

THE BREATHING PROCESS

The act of breathing is a complex muscular performance, whose co-ordination is directed by a respiratory centre in the medulla or hindbrain. Among its nerve cells one group is responsible for inhalation and another for exhalation. Inhalation is an active process; exhalation is a passive process, a recoil or letting go.

The muscles called into action in filling and emptying the lungs are those of the diaphragm, the walls of the chest, and the floating ribs. The diaphragm is the most powerful muscle, acting in a piston-like up-and-down movement. We can see it operating, flattening down and rising again, vigorously in athletes panting after exertion, and gently in a sleeping baby.

During inhalation the dome-shaped diaphragm flattens, pressing down on the ciscera below and bulging out the abdomen in deep breathing; at the same time the thoracic cage expands and the atmospheric pressure outside the body fills the lungs through the nasal passages (or mouth), pharynx, windpipe, and bronchi.

During exhalation, there is a passive recoil. The chest cage relaxes (rather like an umbrella closing), the abdominal wall recoils, and the diaphragm, which was lowered by the pressure of the inflowing air, rises by its own elasticity. During this process, air is expelled from the lungs. Exhalation is a letting-go from the tension of expansion.

Ordinarily, the lungs inflate and deflate some fifteen to twenty times each minute. They have elasticity, but are not muscular organs. They rely for expansion and contraction on the muscles of the thoracic cage and the diaphragm. When the muscles surrounding the lungs expand, a partial vacuum is created, and atmospheric pressure sees to it that air flows into the lungs. The natural elasticity of the lungs and the chest wall, on their recoil, pushes air out of the lungs. The so-called 'iron lung' used in hospitals does not operate by pumping air into the lungs, but by increasing and reducing the air pressure on the outer walls of the chest.

The expansion of the lungs depends on the chest walls providing an air-tight compartment; if the wall is punctured, as in stabbing, air will rush in and collapse the lungs. Occasionally doctors admit air to one side of a patient's chest so as to collapse and rest a diseased lung.

The respiratory centre in the brain operates from nerve feedback information from the lungs and body muscles, and from the oxygen-carbon dioxide balance of the blood passing through the brain. The chemical and nerve controls can be triggered by the emotions, a factor taken into account in Yoga.

RESUSCITATION

Until recently the most widely-used method of artificially stimulating the mechanical process of breathing was to place the patient face downwards, kneel at his side or astride him, facing his head, place one's hands flat against his lower ribs at each side of the spinal column, and then every four or five seconds throw the bodyweight forward onto the hands, between thrusts sitting up and relaxing the pressure without removing the hands from the lower ribs.

But now the most popular method of artificial respiration is mouth-to-mouth, the resuscitator exhaling air from his own lungs into those of the patient, whose head is held back. Air should be transmitted in this way every four or five seconds.

A BEAUTIFUL SYSTEM

Analysis of inhaled and exhaled air shows the former to be composed of 20.95% oxygen, 0.05% carbon dioxide, and 79% nitrogen; and exhaled air of 16.5% oxygen, 4.0% carbon dioxide, and 79.5% nitrogen. Behind these figures is a neat physiological process.

In describing the lungs we mentioned the alveoli, the millions of tiny air sacs, like miniature balloons, around which the blood flows. On an inbreath, by the Law of Gaseous Diffusion, oxygen moves from the area of higher pressure in the air sacs to that of lower pressure in the red blood cells, specifically in the haemoglobin, the colouring matter of the red corpuscles. The blood transports the oxygen to the body cells. The medical term for what then happens is osmosis. Oxygen and nourishment from the food we have eaten, now in liquid form, is handed over to the tissues, and the cells hand over in return their waste (carbon dioxide), which the blood carries back to the lungs. The red blood cells act somewhat like bottles on an assembly line. On their reaching the lungs, the Law of Gaseous Diffusion operates again, but this time with the reverse effect: the pressure of carbon dioxide in the veins being higher, the waste gases move into the air sacs and are expelled from the body on the outgoing breath.

It is a beautiful system, and worth making the most of through Yogic breathing.

RESIDUAL AIR

The air that remains in the body after the bulk has been processed is called the residual volume. Some of this air remains in the lungs, and there is also air in the 'dead space' between the lungs and the nostrils. There can be an increase in the volume of residual air in persons with diseased lungs or in those who have been inactive for a long time. Even the master Yogins must have residual air, but the breathing pauses of *pranayama* are thought to give fresh air the opportunity to diffuse healthfully with static air in the respiratory passages and the lungs.

VITAL CAPACITY

The vital capacity is the maximum volume of air that can be exhaled following a deep breath. Vital capacity for an average person is estimated at 3,800 cubic centimetres, but variations occur due to differences in physical build, or through exercising the muscles of respiration, as in Yoga. The figure of 3,800 cubic centimetres is made up as described below.

In normal breathing at rest the average person takes in about 600 cubic centimetres of air. A further 2,000 cubic centimetres can be drawn in by making an effort to inflate the lungs as fully as possible. 600 cubic centimetres is the average expiration under normal conditions, but this too, with an effort, can be increased by about 1,200 cubic centimetres. Add the three together – they are known respectively as tidal air (600), complemental air (2,000), and supplemental air (1,200) – and we see that the maximum volume of air that can be expelled by this average person (a non-athlete, and untrained in Yogic and other deep breathing) is 3,800 cubic centimetres. This is his vital capacity.

Arthritis and certain other diseases can restrict the capacity of the chest muscles to move, leading to extremely shallow breathing and eventually very often to lung infections. Asthma is a spasm of the bronchial muscle, making exhalation difficult: what is normally a passive act becomes effortful.

OXYGEN DEBT

An oxygen debt occurs when the proportion of oxygen in the bloodstream is less than it should be. A familiar indication of this is a yawn. The debt can be incurred as you read these words by holding your nose firmly for a few seconds. Another indication is that the lungs have to work faster after running or other effortful activity. The amount of carbon dioxide in the bloodstream acts as a trigger: when it exceeds a certain level, a centre in the brain orders faster breathing.

The long-distance runner builds up his oxygen debt slowly. As he runs he breathes more deeply, his heart beats more rapidly, and the exchange of oxygen and carbon dioxide in the body speeds up. But if the long-distance runner has trained properly, this combination of faster and deeper breathing with more rapid blood circulation enables him to cover several miles (in the marathon over twenty-six miles) without great respiratory distress. The sprinter has a somewhat different experience. He makes an all-out effort over a hundred metres. His metabolic demands during this explosive effort are such that there is no natural way of giving the blood cells the oxygen they need: about six quarts in ten seconds or less. So the body makes what might be called a gentleman's agreement with the runner's mind and says: 'All right, run like a hound of hell for a hundred metres, go into oxygen debt for ten seconds or less, and recoup your shortage at the end of the race.' The mind agrees, and the athlete goes 'into the red' for almost the whole requirement of oxygen. But once he has crossed the winning line and pulled up, his mouth is drawn wide open and his lungs dilate and contract like a fast-working bellows until the oxygen debt has been repaid.

So one way to stimulate deeper breathing is to exercise vigorously the body's main muscle masses, as in running or in active sports and games. Another method is that of standing or sitting still and voluntarily breathing deeply. The latter is the way of *pranayama*. Because the large muscles are not worked and because lactic acid does not therefore have to be converted into glycogen in the muscles, this kind of deep breathing is of a different nature to the athletic effort we have just described. The Yogin breathes deeply through a conscious decision that controlled breathing fulfils certain aims.

BREATHE BETTER

Through the practice of *pranayama* the respiratory muscles and the lungs function more effectively, and in a short time this becomes habitual, to the great betterment of psycho-physical well-being. Yogic breathing increases bodily vitality, improves air processing in the lungs, purifies the blood, calms and tones the nervous system, and fosters mental poise and equanimity. It relaxes body and mind.

To dissolve tension, sit poised, back straight, head level; let tension go, open up, and for several minutes breathe smoothly, slowly, and deeply. Influencing the mind through the body muscles is a practical aim which Yoga has made a valuable part of the system. Rhythmic breathing inculcates feelings of lightness and buoyancy felt both in the muscles and in emotional tone. *Pranayama* practice is therefore enjoyable – so much so that one has to guard against going on too long with it, and perhaps inducing giddiness.

The action in shallow breathing is restricted to the upper chest. (Women tend to suffer from shallow breathing more than men.) Only a meagre amount of air enters the lungs, and thus only a small amount of oxygen permeates the blood vessels of the air sacs. Correct breathing enriches the blood, stimulates the circulation, and feeds life-force to the blood, tissues, and organs.

On average the shallow breather is found to inhale about 500 cubic centimetres of air, but the conditioned deep breather can draw in about 4,000 cubic centimetres. Thus deep breathing takes in about eight times as much air as shallow breathing, which fails adequately to aerate the alveoli of the lungs. The air we breathe is composed of approximately 21% oxygen and 79% nitrogen. This oxygen-nitrogen balance is maintained and we cannot increase the proportion of oxygen; but we can improve the ability of the lungs to take in more air and to process air. The volume of air a person can inhale is dependent on the amount of space his chest muscles can create for the lungs to expand into and for them to contract into on the recoil. Running, brisk walking, jogging (alternating running and brisk walking), active sports and games, and deep breathing exercises improve the tone, mobility, elasticity, and strength of the respiratory muscles and increase vital capacity. Vital capacity, as mentioned earlier, is the measured amount of air exhaled in a deep breath. But even in a trained deep breather, vital capacity is only about 75% of the total lung capacity. The condition and sizes of the lungs themselves are factors in the amount of air that can be processed. The sizes of the lungs are normally proportionate to the physical build of the individual.

Dr Kenneth H. Cooper, a major in the United States Air Force Medical Corps, recently led a team which studied the physiological condition of thousands of airmen before and after physical fitness training. The study showed that the trained man can push twenty times his vital capacity through his lungs in one minute, whereas an out-of-condition man has to struggle to force ten times his vital capacity through his lungs. However, six weeks' training was usually enough to enable young airmen who were out of condition to rise from the lower figure to the higher.

Dr Cooper says (102):

Getting oxygen to the body tissues is the rockbottom basis of conditioning, and it's convenient to think of the systems that process and deliver oxygen as one huge, magnificent, wondrous assembly line, complete with receiving lines to dispose of wastes, and the most beautiful engine ever conceived to keep all of it moving.

He also says that conditioning

produces more blood, specifically more hemoglobin which carries the oxygen, more red-blood cells which carry the hemoglobin, more blood plasma which carries the red-blood cells, and consequently more total blood volume. In our laboratory and others, tests have repeatedly shown that men in good physical condition invariably have a larger blood supply than deconditioned men of comparable size. An average-size man may increase his blood volume by nearly a quart in response to aerobic conditioning. And, of this amount, the red cells may increase proportionately more.

SLIMMING

People who take up Yogic breathing may be surprised to find superfluous fat melting away from the waistline, hips, and other places where it is prone to gather. It seems likely that the link between breathing and burning up foodstuffs for energy partly explains this result. *Pranayama* improves metabolic efficiency. The combined practice of *asanas* and *pranayama* also fosters a muscular feeling tone (kinesthesis) that finds the physical effects of overeating uncomfortable and somewhat reprehensible. This too has a bearing on the way Hatha Yoga slims and reshapes the figure. The postures also break up fatty deposits and streamline the body.

WHY WE NEED TO *LEARN* TO BREATHE

That Yoga masters insist we need to learn to breathe correctly puzzles many people. 'What have I been doing with my lungs from the moment of birth?' you may ask. 'Surely the act of breathing is instinctive? I am breathing every minute of my life, am I not?

Otherwise I would be dead in a minute or two. Why, then, should I be told to "learn" to breathe?'

The Yoga master replies something like this: 'Of course you have been breathing all your days. But there is a world of difference between breathing shallowly and incorrectly and breathing well for health and vitality. Left to our natural animal instinct, it is true that we would breathe efficiently: after all, we nearly all manage to do so when babies. But Man is both animal and something more. His glory, and most of his problems likewise, dwell in this mystery of his being naked ape plus much more – one foot solidly on earth, but the other itching to stride the heavens, god-like. Animals in their natural habitat instinctively select those foods which are good for them. Can the same be said of Man? And when it comes to the most fundamental act of all, we find that great numbers of men and women, through faulty and shallow breathing habits, fail to gain the maximum benefit in purification and vitality freely available from the air they inhale.

'The quality of your breathing as a baby – deep, abdominal, relaxed – is almost certain to have been superior to what it is now. Inhibitions and restraints, moral, social, physical (poor posture and bands of muscular tension), and environmental (stuffy rooms and so on) all destroy the growing child's ability to breathe deeply and healthfully. Without our being aware of it, the passing of the years is often accompanied by a deterioration in the efficiency and effectiveness of respiration. Western society, based on competition and results-orientated, contracts the respiratory muscles, and lack of exercise after the end of the schooldays exacerbates a loss of mobility and elasticity in the thoracic muscles and the diaphragm. Breathing becomes shallower and more restricted, resulting in the drawing in of less air and less oxygen, the most vital of all foods.

'Yes, you are breathing now – breathing in a way. You are getting by. You are managing to survive. But if you train yourself to breathe healthfully, Yogic style, you will soon discover that the way you breathed before was a travesty of the real thing, shallow and inadequate. Now you are being asked to breathe *correctly*. Through controlled Yoga breathing you will raise your level of vitality, clarify consciousness, tone your nervous system, brighten your eyes, put bounce in your step, feel light and buoyant, and float along with the flow of life, in harmony with Nature and the Universal Energies.'

SURELY CONTROLLED BREATHING IS UNNATURAL?

The answer to this question is 'No', because the human organism is equipped for both automatic and consciously-regulated breathing. If anything is unnatural, it is the kind of inferior, inadequate breathing habits so often acquired once the carefree years of early childhood have passed.

AUTOMATIC CONTROL

Co-ordination of the act of breathing is operated from a respiratory centre in the medulla or hindbrain. This collection of nerve cells has two parts, one part being responsible for inhalation and the other part for exhalation. The centre operates on the basis of nervous feedback information from the lungs and muscles, and from the oxygen-carbon dioxide balance of the blood passing through the brain. This is automatic machinery on which we depend for staying alive. Yet, unlike most physiological processes, we can also exercise some degree of voluntary control. This also is a necessity for survival, as when we hold our breath under water.

Inspiration comes from an impulse through the vagus nerves and expiration from its inhibition. Inhalation of air is thus an active process, and exhalation a passive process – a recoil or letting go.

Inflating the lungs stretches the sensory nerve endings, a signal for the expiratory part of the respiratory centre in the brain to inhibit the action of inspiration through an impulse along the vagus nerves. When exhalation ends, the vagus action returns, and the in-and-out flow of the life breath continues.

A slight rise in the content of carbon dioxide in the blood results in an immediate command from the respiratory centre for more air to be drawn into the lungs, and the muscular activity necessary for inspiration is triggered off. A gentle example of this is an involuntary yawn; a vigorous example is the panting of the sprinter at the end of a race. A progressive accumulation of carbon dioxide in the body leads to convulsions and an agonizing death. A fall in oxygen, on the other hand, leads to a slow loss of consciousness.

When the haemoglobin is insufficiently oxidized, the blood takes on a bluish tinge. This may occur because heart disease has slowed down the circulation; through lung disease; or because of a low oxygen content in the atmosphere at high altitudes.

Overbreathing when at rest so successfully removes carbon dioxide that respiration may actually cease for several minutes.

CONSCIOUS CONTROL

Along with these automatic functions we have been describing, there is also a measure of voluntary control of breathing. By means of this dual control, Man achieves many of the things that make him distinctively human.

'Considering that our life depends upon our breathing, it is remarkable that we have as much conscious control over it as we do,' says Benjamin F. Miller and Ruth Goode in *Man and His Body* (114).

Our automatic controls keep us breathing, fortunately, whether or not we are paying attention, or we would not be able to go to sleep. If we had only automatic controls, we would not perform many of our most highly developed acts of skill. Nor would we be capable of those most human forms of expression, laughter, song, and speech. (Animals make their sounds by the same physiological mechanisms, but the controls are instinctual or reflex rather than voluntary. . . .)

Probably our survival, or rather the survival of our evolutionary forebears, also depended upon a thousand unforeseen adaptations and co-ordinations in attack and defence that were more skilfully managed with the breath held or expelled at will. And so we have the wonderful gift of dual control, part voluntary, part automatic, of the very breath of life.

Breath control is brought to its most extraordinary development, though not one we should seek to emulate, in burial alive, success in which depends on slowing down the heartbeat by conscious control and surviving on a modicum of air in a trance state. If levitation is possible, it also must be based on breath control. Fully authenticated is the art of engendering body heat through breath control (*tumo*). By this means Yogins in the Himalayas and in Tibet sit for hours, naked or scantily clad, in sub-zero temperatures.

Levitation, burial alive, and *tumo* will be discussed further in a later chapter. It is more important to move on now to a more practical function of the 'wonderful gift of dual control' we all possess – as regulator of the four stages of the act of breathing.

VI Yogic Breath Control

THE FOUR STAGES OF BREATHING

In *pranayama* one is aware that the act of breathing has four distinct stages. We normally think in terms of only two, inhalation and exhalation, forgetting the brief pauses after each before we change gear and go into reverse, as it were.

The four stages are:

i. Inhalation, or puraka. *This in Yoga is a continuous process, evenly controlled.*

ii. A pause in breathing, called kumbhaka, *retaining the air in the inflated lungs. When distinguishing this from stage iv, which is a pause on empty lungs, we will call this stage full pause. B. K. S. Iyengar calls it* antara kumbhaka (33), *and Archie Bahm calls it* abhyantara kumbhaka (65).

iii. Exhalation, or rechaka. *Again, this should be a smooth and continuous process, a recoil or letting go from the inflation of the lungs, the expansion of the thoracic cage, and the pressing down of the diaphragm. In Yoga special care is taken to make sure outbreathing is thorough.*

iv. A pause in breathing again, this time on empty lungs. This is an effortless breath suspension (kumbhaka), *at the end of which a slow smooth inflow of air through the nostrils commences, and we return to stage i. Archie Bahm calls stage iv* bahya kumbhaka (5).

In *pranayama* there is a measured timing ratio for the stages, especially for the first three stages. This ratio is carefully observed. We will return shortly to this matter of timing; meanwhile we will discuss the stages in more detail.

INHALATION (*PURAKA*)

In Yogic breathing this consists of the muscular action detailed earlier when describing the act of breathing. The movement has two parts, working together. In the first part the thoracic cage expands to make room for the lungs to inflate. In the second part the dome-shaped diaphragm flattens out and descends, swelling out the abdomen and, incidentally, massaging beneficially the abdominal viscera.

At this point it needs to be pointed out that Yogic breathing is not a competition to see how much air we can cram into our lungs. Competition is alien to the spirit of Yoga, and here it could be dangerous. The criterion should always be *comfort*. Breathe deeply, pour air into the lungs – but the point at which the inflation and expansion ends should be just before the point at which discomfort intrudes. If you sit easily, with the back straight and the head level, the respiratory muscles will be free to expand and recoil in comfortable *pranayama*.

False reasoning is behind the temptation to cram the lungs with air. For it is a mistake to think that beyond a certain point (which is a comfortable threshold, easily attained), the more air you take in the more oxygen you will absorb, to the benefit of the billions of. body cells. The fact is that a point is reached after a short period of deep breathing when optimal oxygen is being received, and a surplus is then exhaled on the outgoing breath. If the deep breathing follows intense physical activity – as in running a sprint race – then huge amounts of oxygen will be needed and the chest will automatically heave and the mouth gape and gasp for air. But the immobile sitting Yogin is at the opposite end of the activity scale from the sprinter. Though vital capacity is improved, other factors than quantity of air are the Yogin's prime concerns: smoothness, and the length of inspiration and expiration and the in-between pauses. In a word: *control*. The minimum amount of air needed in Yogic practice is during the quiescence of meditation.

SUSPENSION (*KUMBHAKA*)

Holding the breath is a conscious act which checks the mechanism, described earlier, whereby our respiration is automatically regulated. We explained then that inspiration comes from an impulse through the vagus nerves and expiration from its inhibition, and that inflating the lungs stretches the sensory nerve endings, a signal for the expiratory part of the respiratory centre in the brain to inhibit the action of inspiration through an impulse along the vagus nerves. At the end of exhalation, the vagus action returns.

Now, with conscious suspension of breathing, we are switching from 'automatic' to 'manual', as it were. This requires some practice for smoothness and ease. And this means, as mentioned in discussing inhalation above, refraining from forcing, and making comfort the criterion. When *kumbhaka* follows filling the lungs, the thoracic 'umbrella' must stay open and the diaphragm down and the abdomen out during the immobile breathing pause. One has to inhibit an initial tendency of the ribs and diaphragm to recoil during the full pause, and to expand and rise respectively during the empty pause. However, after some weeks of training, inhibition becomes effortless as long as *kumbhaka* is not prolonged to a point of strain.

Once you have supplied the body richly with oxygen through deep breathing – the Yogin, unlike the athlete, is not making excessive calls for supply – you will find that the breath can be held longer without discomfort. In advanced practice Yogins may check their breathing for several minutes, but it would be prudent for most practitioners to suspend breathing for only a few seconds. Experiment will disclose your comfortable limits. The longer you have been breathing deeply, the more relaxed and poised is your sitting position, the more easily will air be retained in the lungs or and empty pause be sustained.

If after retention the air bursts out noisily, the suspension has been over-prolonged: the air should be released in a steady smooth stream from the nostrils. Similarly, following the empty pause, the air should unhurriedly and quietly begin its ascent of the nostrils. Do not push the muscles and lungs beyond comfortable capacity. The ease and comfort of performance should be reflected in the serenity of the facial expression.

During *kumbhaka* with full lungs or empty lungs, one should resist the temptation to let a little air through the nostrils or mouth to keep the suspension going comfortably. The abdomen should not change tone by contracting or relaxing.

THE IMPORTANCE OF SUSPENSION

Every day we perform numerous little *kumbhakas;* but few people give any thought to how much control of breathing is tied up with the diurnal pursuit of being a human. We suspend breathing to listen intently; to concentrate; to cry, sob, laugh, sing; when we are surprised; when we are waiting 'with bated breath'; when we need to be very still or very silent.

But what does Yogic breath suspension achieve? Why is it so important in *pranayama?*

There are esoteric answers, connected with the arousal and channelling of latent inner powers: but this aspect will be discussed in a later section of this book. The direct benefits from *kumbhaka* are both physiological and psychological.

A possible physiological benefit from *kumbhaka* is that the pause gives time for a better mixing of fresh air with the stale residual air in the air sacs of the lungs. The fact that some residual air remains in the 'dead space' between the nostrils and the bronchi and in the lungs was mentioned several pages back, in our account of the anatomy and physiology of respiration. Several writers on Hatha Yoga have pointed out that a suspension of breathing on filled lungs can have a cleansing and purifying effect on residual air. One of these is Professor Ernest Wood. The figures for residual air vary somewhat according to which textbook one consults, but the principle Professor Wood posits remains valid (91):

While the inflow and outflow of air should be 'regular', still an occasional practice of inner suspension (*kumbhaka*) has a cleansing value. We can see how this works, especially with reference to the alveolar air in the lungs. The lungs may be considered in three parts – the wider channels (the bronchi), then the narrower passages (the bronchioles), and lastly the very fine, even hair-fine, clusters of branchlets (the alveoli). A standard intake of breath by the average person occupies approximately two seconds. If it is 'shallow' it does not satisfactorily aerate the alveoli. Now, shallowness is not a matter of time or length of the inhalation, but of lack of strength and decisive action of the chest muscles, so that there is here an important point to be considered by shallow breathers, and to be acted upon by means of some decisive muscle-toning and habit-forming exercise. . . .

It must be understood that after full expiration the lungs are by no means empty of air. There will be, let us say, in a given person (for cases differ) 150 cubic centimetres of air in the space from the nostril to and including the bronchioles, which is termed 'dead space' because the air therein does not penetrate the relatively thick walls and produce any interchange of gases with the blood. After the expiration there will be, say, 200 cubic centimetres of air remaining in the lungs. Now, in inhaling let us say that 500 cubic centimetres of new air comes in, 150 cubic centimetres of the mixture will still be in the 'dead space', and 350 cubic centimetres will join the unexpired alveolar air, which is higher in carbon dioxide content and lower in oxygen content than the incoming air. A standard figure is that inhaled air contains 21% oxygen and exhaled air about 12%. The aeration of the blood is a big business, since the whole of the blood flows through the lungs in about 3 minutes, and amounts to one fifth of the entire weight of the body.

It is in the manner in which this incoming air arrives in the aureoles that one finds reason for the *kumbhaka* exercise. Experiments have been made which indicate that the diffusion or mixing of the inspired air (with its higher oxygen content and its lower carbon dioxide content) with the static air takes a little time. Further, the new air enters in the form of a cone in the centre of the duct, so that the old air still forms a layer on the inside walls of the tube until that diffusion takes place. . . .

I take it that the *kumbhaka* allows of more perfect diffusion than would occur when the exhalation begins immediately at the cessation of the inhalation. The ratio of inbreathing (1 unit of time), holding (4 units), and outbreathing (2 units) which is generally followed and taught by the *hatha-yogis* must, however, have been arrived at empirically, with a view to maximum benefit and operational economy, although it is thus seen to be scientifically sound.

In advanced Yoga practice 1:4:2 is indeed the timing ratio followed, but it must be understood at this point that 1:1:1 or 1:1:2 is a more realistic and less potentially harmful timing for the beginner or intermediate student. We will come to the timing of inspiration, retention, and expiration shortly.

'All forms of Yoga aim at producing a state of tranquillity in the subject,' says Aubrey Menen in *The New Mystics*. Yogins speak of *kevala kumbhaka*. *Kevala* means 'perfect', 'pure', 'whole'. *Kevala kumbhaka* refers to the practice of respiratory pause, either at the end of inbreathing or outbreathing, when it has become effortless and refined, so that the experience is one of inner peace and tranquillity, a freedom from anxiety, fear, and negative emotions of all kinds, at its highest 'the peace that passeth all understanding'. The benefits of repeated short peaceful respiratory pauses in *pranayama* is cumulative. The nervous system is soothed and calmed, and something of the tranquillity of Yoga practice is carried into everyday living. Combined with the postures, with mind-stilling meditation, and with the many other techniques of Yoga, breath regulation and breath suspension make their large contribution to conducing to equanimity of mind, in Sanskrit *samatwa*. To paraphrase Mr Menen, all techniques of Yoga aim at producing a state of tranquillity in the subject.

LOCKS (*BANDHAS*)

Various muscular restraints, seals, or locks are employed in advanced *pranayama*. The Sanskrit term is *bandha*, related etymologically to the English 'band', 'bind', 'bond', and 'bound'. *Bandhas* are part of a larger grouping called *mudras*, which are muscle controls or exercises devised for special attainments, usually of an esoteric nature, and for more specific results than the general postures (*asanas*). There are 'seals' relating only to the control of energy currents within the body – such as *mula bandha* and *asvini mudra*, which are associated with the sexual energies, and the bizarre *khechari mudra*, which requires that the tongue be cut loose from its attachment to the floor of the mouth, so as to be free to curl back and block off the passage of air from the nostrils to the windpipe. These esoteric controls will be brought up again later, but a few locks employed in holding the breath steady will be described now – though in my opinion their use is best put to suspending breathing for durations in excess of the moderate *kumbhakas* advocated in our practical approach. The reason I say this is that each in some way creates muscular tensions and pressures that disturb the sense of lightness, buoyancy, and psycho-physical freedom that should be an exhilarating and liberating reward of Yogic breathing. It is true that they are recommended in a number of works on Hatha Yoga, including some written for the popular market. Readers may wish to experiment, and some may find the locks useful and without the discomfort experienced by this writer, who admittedly has a dislike of unnecessary restraints and muscular tensions. The use of the muscular locks is conceded if you are holding the breath for longer than, say, one minute – an exact time is impossible to give, for individual capacities vary. In advanced practice breath suspension may be sustained for several minutes, with profuse sweating and trembling; locking is then clearly essential. But our practical approach does not include *pranayama* carried to such lengths.

Stopping air from entering the nostrils requires some practice. Some people acquire the ability to pinch the nostrils by mental control, and also to dilate them to inhale air. Closing the mouth is a primary seal, and should be employed by all readers; this is combined with keeping the air steady in the lungs and in the passages ('dead spaces') between the nostrils and the lungs. This air can be used as a kind of 'ball' (metaphorically, not literally) to block any intrusion of external air into the body. A further control is essential: the muscles of respiration – the thoracic cage, the diaphragm, the abdomen – must, like the air in the lungs and passages, be held immobile.

The technique just described this writer finds adequate, but other methods are suggested in Yogic literature, and these some readers at least may wish to try out. Each, as mentioned above, involves some kind of muscular contraction or pressure.

One of these techniques is to lift the soft palate against the roof of the pharynx. Another is to close the glottis. Whether you know what the glottis is or not, you use it every time you swallow, and it can be dilated at will to modulate the tones of the voice. Italian operatic tenors sometimes employ what is known as the glottal stop to give a high note a cutting edge and a faintly explosive effect – the great Caruso was not immune from this gimmick. We have reflexes that command the glottis to open again after each swallow, so that the trick of keeping the glottis closed for some seconds has to be worked on. It is achieved by starting to swallow, and then freezing the movement at the point when the trachea or windpipe has closed.

Both the techniques described in the preceding paragraph I find unpleasant, imposing a suffocating feeling that defeats the purpose. Some readers, however, may find either one or both of the techniques helpful and not uncomfortable. But I repeat, in moderate *kumbhaka* bodily immobility plus the 'ball of air' method described above should prove adequate and have no tension-producing drawbacks. However, the two most frequently recommended *bandhas* have yet to be described. Their use in prolonged *kumbhaka* is

probably essential, though not, I say again, in moderate breath
suspension.

Chin Lock (Jalandhara Bandha)
Jala means 'a net'. The neck is stretched up and the chin lowered
until it is pressing into the jugular notch between the collar bones
and high up on the breastbone. The position is very similar to the
one you should have already experience in performing the Shoulderstand. In that posture you could not do otherwise, for the chest is
brought against the chin in elevating the legs, pelvis, and trunk to a
candle-straight vertical. But in the Shoulderstand one should always
breathe as freely as possible, whereas *Jalandhara Bandha* is a way
of firmly suspending breathing.

As with the soft palate and glottal controls, I experience a
constricted and suffocating feeling during the Chin Lock. B. K. S.
Iyengar considers *Jalandhara Bandha* essential; otherwise, he says,
pressure is felt on the heart, behind the eyeballs, and in the ears,
and the head feels dizzy. This may be so for prolonged breath
control, but my experience is the reverse in moderate *kumbhaka*,
when the contraction of the throat and neck causes a build-up of
pressure. I am not alone in feeling this, for other students of Yoga
report similar experiences; and my experience agrees with that of
Archie Bahm, who finds the Chin Lock more valuable in sustaining
a pause on emptied lungs than on filled lungs. He says (5): 'This
position proves more useful in holding an empty pause, for the
pressure of the chin against the chest pushes the base of the tongue
and the larynx up into the pharynx and against the palate, thus
providing aid in resisting the pressure caused by the vacuum in the
lungs.' This account of what happens during *Jalandhara Bandha*
reveals why I experience a choking effect and discomfort in the
Chin Lock similar to that in lifting the soft palate against the roof
the pharynx or in closing the glottis. It may be, of course, that
persisting with practice of any of these three methods would eventually lead to a dissolving of my discomfort and psychological
resistance.

Abdominal Uplift (Uddiyana Bandha)
Uddiyana means 'flying up'. This muscle control was described
earlier. The lungs are emptied, the diaphragm is drawn up into the
cavity of the thorax, and the abdominal wall and viscera are pulled

back towards the spine, creating a deep hollow. The diaphragm is immobilized and a lock put on breathing action until the diaphragm and abdominal wall are released. The lock applies only to the empty pause, and clearly would be harmful on full lungs. Deep retraction is possible only on a full exhalation and an empty stomach. An instroke of the abdomen expels air and would be counterproductive following an inhalation. *Uddiyana* and the Chin Lock can be combined effectively.

Abdominal Uplift is effective for its purpose on emptied lungs, but it is based on a muscular contraction and it is not necessary for breath suspension of moderate duration. A drawback to its use, in my opinion, is the difficulty of releasing smoothly the retraction of the abdominal wall and diaphragm following a breath suspension: a sharp recoil causes an involuntary jerked inrush of air into the nostrils, whereas in skilled *pranayama* there should be a smooth, gentle start to inhalation or exhalation. Here again, some readers may not find this a problem.

Uddiyana Bandha is included among the cleansing processes in the classic texts, for reasons given in the section on that aspect of Yoga practice. We repeat what we said then - that the Abdominal Uplift is a superb muscle control in its own right, massaging and toning the diaphragm, abdominal wall, and abdominal organs (viscera), and is probably the greatest discovery ever made for achieving and maintaining intestinal and abdominal health and stimulating peristaltic action in the intestines, leading to more efficient absorption of nourishment from food and to regular natural emptying of the bowels.

The expression 'flying up' has also an esoteric reference. *Prana* or cosmic energy 'flies up' the main *nadi* or subtle nerve of the astral or subtle body. We will return to this in a later section.

In very advanced *pranayama*, *kumbhaka* may be prolonged for several minutes, until the subject sweats profusely, trembles, and even (we are told in the *Siva Samhita*) starts making short hops on the buttocks along the ground. When breath suspension is pursued to such lengths, suitable locks and seals are obviously essential.

WARNING

No more than momentary pauses between inhalation and exhalation are safe for persons with lung, heart, eye, or ear troubles, or for persons with high blood pressure. Inhalations and exhalations should be only of moderate length, and the vigorous breathing exercises, the Cleansing Breath and the Bellows Breath described below, should be omitted. Persons with low blood pressure may pause briefly after breathing in, but should make no deliberate pause after breathing out. The breath should not be deliberately held during pregnancy.

If you have any doubts as to the suitability of any breath control, consult your doctor.

EXHALATION (*RECHAKA*)

In *pranayama*, usually twice as much time is allocated to emptying the lungs as to filling them – a result of the importance given to thorough exhalation in traditional Yoga.

Carbon dioxide, the waste product which the cells exchange for fresh oxygen every three minutes, is expelled from the body on the outgoing breath. Some residual air, as we have seen, remains; but the more complete and efficient the exhalation, the more efficient the purification, and the greater the lung expansion and inflow of fresh air and oxygen on the following inspiration.

The Austrian psychotherapist Wilhelm Reich, a pupil of Sigmund Freud, found that his neurotic patients had developed muscular blockages against thorough expulsion of stale air. The ability of persons who have advanced far in Yogic self-mastery to respond calmly in situations which would before have evoked an excited response – anxiety, anger, flight, or fight – is in large part due to mastery over breathing. Yoga psychology says that all ideas have attendant emotions and that these play upon the respiratory processes. Excited emotions mean jerky breathing; smooth breathing means calm emotions. Reich's work confirms this.

Full exhalation is a central technique in the psychotherapy of the Reichian School. Reich himself wrote (116):

> There is no neurotic individual who is capable of exhaling in one breath, deeply and evenly. The patients have developed all conceivable practices which prevent *deep expiration*. They exhale 'jerkily', or, as soon as the air is let out, they quickly bring their chests back into the inspiratory position. Some patients describe the inhibition, when they

become aware of it, as follows: 'It is as if a wave of the ocean struck
a cliff. It does not go on.'

The sensation of this inhibition is localized in the upper abdomen
or in the middle of the abdomen. With deep expiration, there appear
in the abdomen vivid sensations of pleasure or anxiety. The function
of the respiratory block (inhibition of deep expiration) is exactly that
of avoiding the occurrence of these sensations. As a preparation for the
process of bringing about the orgasm reflex, I ask my patients to
'follow through' with their breathing, to 'get into swing'. If one asks
the patients to breathe deeply, they usually force the air in and out in
an artificial manner. This voluntary behaviour serves only to prevent
the natural vegetative rhythms of respiration. It is unmasked as an
inhibition; the patient is asked to breathe without effort, that is, *not to
do breathing exercises*, as he would like to do. After five to ten breaths,
respiration usually becomes deeper and the first inhibitions make their
appearance. With *natural* deep expiration, the head moves *spontaneously* backwards at the end of expiration. Patients are unable to let
their heads go back in this spontaneous manner. They stretch their
heads forward in order to prevent this spontaneous backward movement, or they jerk their heads violently to one side or the other side;
at any rate, the movement is different from that which would come
about naturally.

With natural respiration, the shoulders become relaxed and move
gently and slightly forward at the end of expiration. Our patients hold
their shoulders tight just at the end of expiration, pull them up or
back; in brief, they execute various shoulder movements in order not
to let the spontaneous vegetative movement come to pass.

TIMING

Yogic breathing is based on rhythm, and rhythm is life.

Strain can be avoided by keeping to a ratio between inhalation,
retention, and exhalation of 1:1:1 for beginners, and later of 1:1:2.
A few people may care to go on, whenever it is comfortable, to
1:2:2, but I do not recommend, without long preparation and
personal supervision, the traditional ratio of 1:4:2.

Start breathing again after retention immediately the onset of any
strain is discerned – at the first faint warning tickle, like the intima-
tion of a sneeze; but in normal practice you should resume breathing

action a little before that point. There are sound commensense grounds for sticking to 1:1:1 or 1:1:2; and the person who thinks that increasing the duration of breath retention will bestow on him occult powers is playing a dangerous game.

If you are unable to practise breathing with evenness, you need to shorten the duration of the stages. Remember that evenness of breathing is conducive to evenness of mind.

Few Yoga instructors teach more than a brief pause on empty lungs. The timing ratio quoted in Yoga literature is nearly always three figures rather than four. Archie Bahm (5) is an exception, for he considers that a longer empty pause is conducive to relaxation.

Counting seconds silently is the most straightforward method of timing. Some practice at inwardly repeating 'one'; 'two'; 'three'; or 'hundred-and-one'; 'hundred-and-two'; 'hundred-and-three;' and so on, with a watch before you, matching up the count with the seconds, will produce a skill useful in *pranayama* and also in activities outside Yoga. (I have always used it, with no loss of efficiency, in timing photographic enlargement exposures, and have never purchased a darkroom clock.)

Another method of timing is to repeat silently the Sanskrit words for inspiration, suspension, and expiration – *puraka, kumbhaka*, and *rechaka*. To accord with a 1:1:2 ratio, one would therefore silently pronounce '*puraka*' once, '*kumbhaka*' once, and '*rechaka*' twice as the basic timing units. Each word, it is true, has three syllables, but Sanskrit words do not come easily to Western lips and it can be embarrassing to compare your own pronunciation with that of an Indian.

Some Yogins listen to and count their heartbeats, but this is a technique not everyone can acquire.

There is another traditional method which uses a *matra* as the measure. Vachaspati, in his gloss on the *Yoga Sutras* of Patanjali, says: 'A *matra* is the time which is taken up by thrice turning up one's hand over one's knee and then snapping the fingers once. Measured by thirty-six such *matras* is the first attempt (*udghata*), which is mild. Twice that is the second, which is middling. Thrice that is the third, which is intense. This is the *Pranayama* as measured by number.' Theos Bernard says that a *matra* 'is generally considered to be equivalent to our second.'

Learning to count seconds silently seems the most practical approach.

SITTING FOR YOGIC BREATHING

The postures of Hatha Yoga, by stretching the muscles and by toning, relaxing, and strengthening the muscles of the chest, diaphragm, and abdomen, and improving their mobility and elasticity, encourage deep and efficacious breathing. The nature of many of the *asanas* is to trigger off naturally deep abdominal breathing. Stretching stimulates circulation and respiration, and by lifting bands of tension from the chest, diaphragm, and abdomen, sets free the muscles of deep breathing. Smooth deep breathing is an integral part of the performance of many postures.

But for Yogic breathing proper (*pranayama*) an immobile poised sitting posture is invariably adopted. This means sitting cross-legged on the floor with the back kept straight, the head held level, and the head, neck, and backbone in a vertical line, though always without rigidity. The sitting postures used for *pranayama* are the same as those used for meditation. Here, for Yogic breathing, we must be able to sit easily and without movement (other than respiratory) for fifteen minutes.

The experienced Yogin probably will sit in either the Perfect Posture or the Lotus Posture, both of which were described in the section on the *asanas*. But beginners may use the Easy Posture, which is as simple as its name implies. If you carried out the advice to start using it as soon as it was described earlier in this book, by now you will probably be able to sustain it comfortably for fifteen minutes of breath regulation. If not, sit with the head and spine in a vertical line on a straight-backed chair, or on a stool with your back and the back of your head against a wall.

When the head, neck, and spine are kept in poised vertical line, the internal organs are not cramped in any way: the ribs are free to expand and recoil to their limit of mobility, the lungs have space to inflate and deflate within the thoracic cage, and the abdomen is free of pressures either from below or from above, so long as no tight clothing, belt or girdle is worn. The diaphragm, between the thoracic cage and the abdomen, is unconstrained in performing its natural piston-like down-and-up action during inhalation and exhalation respectively. There is a sense of freedom and poise, and deep smooth *pranayama* is closely associated with both.

HAND POSITIONS

You can cup your hands in your lap, the back of the top hand resting on the palm of the hand below, the thumbs touching; or rest the right palm on the right knee and the left palm on the left knee. But if you wish to observe good traditional form, you should straighten the arms until they are locked at the elbows and rest the back of the left wrist on the left knee and the back of the right wrist on the right knee. Hold your fingers in the Symbol or Seal of Knowledge (*Jnana Mudra*), which means bringing the tips of the thumbs and forefingers together and holding the other fingers out straight. The index finger here symbolizes the individual spirit (*Atman*) and the thumb the cosmic spirit (*Brahman*). The gesture thus represents the Union that is Yoga.

The only break from these positions is when one hand is raised to manipulate the nostrils with the fingers during the Alternate Nostril Breath. This technique is described and illustrated in the account of that exercise.

HOW OFTEN, AND FOR HOW LONG?

If you join an *ashram* in India you may be expected to practise *pranayama* four times a day: soon after rising in the morning, at noon, in the early evening, and shortly before retiring to bed for a night's sleep. But here we recommend once a day, morning or evening, or twice a day if you are very keen, morning *and* evening. If you practise once a day devote fifteen to twenty minutes to *pranayama*, and if twice a day, give ten minutes on each occasion.

PRE-REQUIREMENTS

Certain commonsense pre-requirements need to be observed before starting a session of breath controls.

Practise *pranayama* at a different time from postures. There should be an interval of at least one hour between finishing breath controls and starting postures, or between finishing postures and starting *pranayama*. There are several good reasons for this separation of the two programmes. Deep rhythmic breathing is an integral part of the postures, and you spend the whole of the fifteen minutes of Yogic breathing sitting in one of the postures. If combined, the programmes could produce fatigue by the end, instead of the customary refreshment. Moreover, starting the postures with the lungs highly ventilated and the organism highly vitalized is not the ideal approach: in some *asanas*, such as the inverted poses, it could produce dizziness. And, lastly, joining the two programmes together makes it more difficult to sustain the special kind of awareness and total attention that Yoga exercise requires.

Allow at least two hours to pass after a main meal, and one hour after a light snack, before starting *pranayama*.

Sit in a clean, well-ventilated, pleasant room; better still, sit out of doors when the weather and temperature permit.

Wear a minimum of slackly-fitting clothing, or no clothing at all if conditions permit, so enabling your skin to join fully in the breathing.

Empty the bladder just before practice and evacuate the bowels if you can. The former is always possible; the latter can be achieved regularly if you make a habit of going to stool at this time every day.

Pranayama is a process of purification. It is traditional before breathing practice to wash the hands and face with tepid or cold water, to gargle and rinse out the mouth, and to massage the tongue and gums gently with the fingers for a minute or so. Some Yogins also clean the tongue by scraping it carefully and gently with the back of a spoon.

Blow each nostril sharply a few times to clear it. One nostril is likely to remain partly blocked, but opens further during exercise. Some Yogins use the traditional nasal cleansing method of drawing water up the nostrils and expelling it from the mouth: this clears the nostrils and is said to prevent colds, though not everyone finds it easy to become accustomed to the strange sensation.

According to Hatha Yoga teaching, the flow of *prana* normally changes from one nostril to the other every two hours, and one nostril is usually partially or totally closed. You can clear a nostril by lying on that side with the arm strongly pressed against the body, or alternatively by pressing down the armpit on the active side on top of a chair-back or a similar narrow firm object. The Hatha Yogins actually use a piece of equipment which looks rather like a crutch for this purpose; the lower end rests firmly on the ground and the Yogin presses down his armpit on the handle.

PERFORMANCE

Sit in one of the meditative cross-legged postures or on a straight-backed chair or a stool with your back against a wall. Head and backbone must be in a straight vertical line.

Close the eyes to help the mind focus sharply on the breath flow. In the stable sitting posture there should be no overbalancing or swaying.

Breathe through the nostrils, not the mouth, unless instructed to the contrary in the description of the exercise. Yogins point out that the mouth is for eating and the nostrils are for breathing. Blood circulating in the nasal passages heats the inhaled air so that it is warmed before entering the lungs. The nostrils also perform two more valuable services: dry air is moistened in the passages, and the hairs in the nostrils trap dust or any foreign matter in the atmosphere that could be harmful if it reached the lungs. Many Yogins develop an ability to dilate the nostrils to produce a silent and automatic inflow of air.

Never force any of the stages of breathing. Especially is this true of suspending the breath (*kumbhaka*). Never cram the lungs with air to what feels like almost bursting point. Start the breath flowing again before reaching the point of discomfort or strain in the suspension.

If the tongue is kept still, saliva should not be a problem; but if it does gather, you should swallow it, though not while holding the breath or exhaling it.

Powerful practice causes profuse sweating and muscular trembling, but this should rarely result from the moderate practice advised here. If it does, bring the session to an end with a few minutes relaxation, lying on the back in the Corpse Posture.

There is a right attitude of mind for performing Yogic breathing, and that is one of calmness, quietness, and total attention. Concentration is complete, yet never effortful. The Buddhists call such rapt and effortless attention 'mindfulness'. When turned to *pranayama*, one becomes unsure whether one is directing a breathing activity or being breathed, just as brilliant ballroom dancers cease to be conscious of which of them is the leader and which the led.

Some treatises advise harnessing the considerable powers of the imagination during breath controls, visualizing the expulsion of fatigue toxins and impurities on exhalation, and the intake of purity, oxygen, vitality, and *prana* on the inhalation.

PREPARATIONS FOR THE TRADITIONAL *PRANAYAMAS*

The inadequacies of shallow high upper-chest breathing have already been stressed, and so has the importance of breathing deeply and diaphragmatically. It was also explained how the diaphragm, the key and largest muscle in the act of breathing, acts like a piston, flattening out and moving down on inhalation, and rising and regaining its dome shape on exhalation. With each inspiration and expiration during deep breathing there is a concomitant action on the abdominal wall, which swells out on the inspiration and subsides and moves back towards the spine on the expiration. It is important to experience this combined diaphragmatic and abdominal move-ment, to feel it clearly and to memorize that feeling, and to acquire the habit of deep breathing in this way for life.

Supine Abdominal Breathing
One effective way of acquiring this experience and habit in the early stages of learning is to lie flat on the back, the legs fully extended, the arms bent, and the palms of the hands flat on the abdomen so that the tips of the longest fingers meet over the navel. The backs of the upper arms rest on the floor, and the forearms are held in against the ribs.

Only the thoracic cage, the diaphragm, and the abdomen will be in action, so relax the rest of the body muscles. The full length of the back should be flat against the floor. If the legs are relaxed, the feet should naturally fall out to the side, with the inside edges of the heels staying in contact, or almost so. If the lower back stays down flat on the floor, the muscular sensations of the widening of the thoracic cage will be more strongly felt.

Now inhale slowly, taking a deep unhurried breath, though with-out cramming the lungs with air to the point of discomfort. Con-centrate your attention fully on the muscular movement: the ribs expanding outwards, pushing against the forearms, the diaphragm flattening and moving down, the abdomen swelling out and rising below the palms of the hands (*see* illustration). Breathe slowly and smoothly, through the nostrils, not the mouth.

Pause for two or three seconds at the comfortable limit of inspiration; then start releasing air slowly and steadily from the nostrils. The reverse muscular process to that of inhalation will now be experienced. Note the sensations carefully, as you did during inbreathing. The ribs subside like an umbrella being closed, the forearms move inwards in sympathy with the thoracic cage, the diaphragm rises, the abdomen flattens and moves back towards the spine below the palms of the hands (*see* illustration). Make a thorough exhalation; pause for two or three seconds; then start another inhalation.

Breathe slowly and evenly in this way – inspiration, brief pause, expiration, brief pause, inspiration, and so on – for about three minutes. Give your full attention to memorizing the muscular sensations of deep breathing – the thoracic, diaphragmatic, and abdominal movements, the pressures against the palms of the hands and the forearms, and those of the back against the floor.

After four weeks of daily practice you should record the muscular sensations with the palms of the hands and the forearms only during the first minute of Supine Abdominal Breathing. During the following two minutes keep the palms of the hands flat on the floor and the arms relaxed along the sides of the body, and with muscular (kinesthetic) sense, without the aid of the palms or forearms, concentrate on the now subtler sensations of deep breathing as you slowly and smoothly inhale and exhale. Again take careful mental note of the rise and fall of the abdomen, the down-and-up movement of the diaphragm, and the out-and-in, umbrella-like expansion and recoil of the rib-cage.

One important further operation is necessary. So that deep healthful breathing becomes an established habit, from now on, as long as it proves valuable, for a minute or two several times each day – while standing, sitting, walking, or lying on your back – move the beam of your attention to your breathing and re-create the sensations of abdominal breathing anew.

Pumping
This is a useful associate exercise to Supine Abdominal Breathing. It is an abdominal rather than a breathing exercise, but it focuses attention on the rise and fall of the abdomen, as the preceding

breathing exercise does, though it is more localized and powerful. At the same time it beneficially massages the abdominal viscera.

Lie flat on the back, the arms by the sides with the palms of the hands turned up, the legs fully extended together. Relax fully, and concentrate all your attention on the abdomen – the head, neck, shoulders, arms, and legs all stay relaxed. The back should be flat against the floor along its full length. Take a rapid deep breath through the nostrils, so that the abdominal wall swells out; then immediately pull the abdomen back towards the spine with a sharp instroke and expel air from the nose in an exhalation as rapid as the preceding inhalation. It is important that the shoulders, the upper and lower back, and the pelvis stay in firm contact with the floor. All the action is centred in the abdomen, except for the inevitable piston action of the diaphragm and the expansion and recoil of the rib-cage – but this being an abdominal and not a breathing exercise, all your attention should be brought to bear on the swelling out and pulling in of the abdominal wall.

Each out-and-in movement of the abdomen should take one second, and ten successive out-and-in movements should be performed. Relax for about twenty seconds, breathing normally; then perform another round of Pumping.

Pumping should be performed daily during the period of establishing the habit of abdominal breathing, and may be continued afterwards by those readers who find its deep massage beneficial.

The Complete Yoga Breath
This differs from Supine Abdominal Breathing only in being a fuller sensation, and always being performed with the back and head held erect. You are conscious that you draw more air into the lungs and empty them more thoroughly. The upright posture makes possible a greater vital capacity than is practicable when lying flat on the back. But this should not be taken to mean the filling of every nook and cranny of the lungs, which is physiologically impossible, or the emptying out of every scrap of air from the same organs, which is again physiologically impossible. It does, however, mean an inhalation carried to the point of a feeling of fullness without strain, and an exhalation carried to the point of full subsidence of the abdomen, full raising of the diaphragm, and full recoil of the ribs, accompanied by the feeling of having emptied the lungs completely. *Complete Yoga Breath* is the customary description of this exercise, and only

pedants will cavil at the use of the word 'complete'. The movement is complete in that you are conscious of all the respiratory muscles working and have a feeling first of fullness, and then of emptiness in the lungs.

Sit on the floor in one of the cross-legged postures, or on a straight-backed chair, keeping the back and head erect, the hands cupped in the lap, or right and left hand on right and left knee respectively. Kneeling and then sitting back on the heels with the spine straight and vertical also encourages natural deep breathing. Inhale and exhale through the nostrils.

In the Complete Yoga Breath you fill the lungs to a point of fullness without strain or discomfort. A key part of the 'completeness' of this exercise is to think of the lungs as having three parts – this is a ruse, a visualization, an employment of imagination, but it serves a purpose. Think of the lungs as being composed of lower, middle, and upper spaces. The lower lungs are visualized and imagined as being filled first; then the middle lungs; and finally the upper lungs: the accompanying muscular movements are the act of breathing described above – thoracic cage expanding, diaphragm lowering, abdomen swelling out – divided into three stages, and reaching the limit of expansion at the conclusion of the third stage, filling the upper lungs and broadening the chest. Some instructors advise lifting the collar bones at the very end of the inspiration, in addition to the diaphragmatic and intercostal action. There is a tendency for shallow high-chest breathers to lift their shoulders, and it is therefore undesirable, in my opinion, in daily habit or in practising the Complete Yoga Breath.

The Complete Yoga Breath fills and empties the lungs very efficiently, richly oxygenating the blood during filling and removing waste gases during emptying. Though the exercise is visualized as having three stages, there should be one continuous smooth movement. Do not strain – when the lungs feel comfortably full, stop the movement and the intake of air. Exhale in a controlled smooth continuous movement, the air streaming steadily out of the nostrils. Employ imagination to think of and visualize an inflow of universal energy (*prana*) and an outflow of impurities and fatigue toxins.

Make four or five complete in-and-out breaths in a minute. Rest for twenty seconds, and then perform four or five more Complete Yoga Breaths. Include pauses between inhalation and exhalation, and between exhalation and inhalation, lasting two or three seconds.

The Complete Yoga Breath vitalizes; removes phlegm; tones and steadies the nervous system; purifies and enriches the blood; improves appetite; aids digestion; broadens and strengthens the thorax; massages the abdominal organs; and makes consciousness lucid and alert. Once it has been mastered, deep, even, and rhythmical breathing can be produced at will. It will be found valuable at times when instant vitality is required. It has the power to lift anxious, fearful, and melancholy moods.

Walking Breath Control
Professor Wood (91) suggests that beginners may start regulating respiration by taking a brisk early-morning walk, breathing in for eight paces, and then breathing out for the following eight paces; and that the beginner takes such walks for two weeks to a month before starting *pranayama*.

I see no need for such a preliminary, but recommend Walking Breath Control at any time of day for students at any stage of experience. As the student introduces breath pauses, these can be included in the breathing rhythm of walking also. But avoid excesses. It would not be sensible to employ breath control throughout a walk of several miles: rather, perform five or six in-and-out breaths, and then breathe freely for two or three minutes; then repeat the rhythmic controlled breathing for five or six in-and-out breaths. Three rounds of such regulated breathing will be sufficient for the beginner, increasing gradually to ten on longish walks.

THE TRADITIONAL *PRANAYAMAS*

The preceding controls – Supine Abdominal Breathing and the Complete Yoga Breath – are preparations for the traditional *pranayamas*, eight in number. The *Hatha Yoga Pradipika* says (75):
Brahma and other Devas [gods] were always engaged in the exercise of *Pranayama*, and, by means of it, got rid of the fear of death. Therefore, one should practise *Pranayama* regularly. So long as the breath is restrained in the body, so long as the mind is undisturbed, and so long as the gaze is fixed between the eyebrows, there is no fear from Death. When the system of the *Nadis* becomes clear of the impurities by properly controlling the *prana*, then the air, piercing the entrance of the *Sushumna* [spinal channel], enters it easily. Steadiness of mind

comes when the air moves freely in the middle [of the *Sushumna*]. This is the *manomani* condition [*samadhi*], which is attained when the mind becomes calm. To accomplish it, various *Kumbhakas* are performed by those who are expert in the methods; for, by the practice of different *Kumbhakas*, wonderful success is attained. *Kumbhakas* are of eight kinds, viz. *Surya Bhedana, Ujjayi, Sitkari, Sitali, Bhastrika, Bhramari, Murchha,* and *Plavini.*

The *Gheranda Samhita* says (87): 'The *Kumbhakas* or retentions of breath are of eight sorts; *Sahita, Surya-bheda, Ujjayi, Sitali, Bhastrika, Bharmari, Murchha,* and *Kevali.*' The substitutes *Sahita* and *Kevali* are controls belonging to esoteric *pranayama* and need not concern us now.

To the eight main traditional controls we will here add a ninth, *Kapalabhati,* which is included with the purification (hygienic) practices in the classic texts, but which is now usually listed as *pranayama.*

Cleansing Breath (Kapalabhati)

'When inhalation and exhalation are performed very quickly, like a pair of bellows of a blacksmith, it dries up all the disorders from the excess of phlegm, and is known as *Kapalabhati,*' says the *Hatha Yoga Pradipika* (75). *Kapala* means 'skull' and *bhati* means 'light'. This is the only major Yogic breathing exercise that does not include a breath retention (*kumbhaka*), though the somewhat similar Bellows Breath (*Bhastrika*) includes an apoenia only on the last breath of each round.

Kapalabhati is one of the *shatkarmas* or purifying techniques, and its purpose is not deep breathing but a cleansing of the frontal air passages. It should therefore be performed immediately before practice of the main *pranayamas.* The Bellows Breath (*Bhastrika*) may be used as a substitute, and is slightly more vigorous.

To perform *Kapalabhati,* you breath in and out rapidly, contracting the stomach muscles and pulling them back towards the spine on each sharp expulsion of air, and immediately letting go from the contraction so that the natural recoil of the abdominal wall brings an automatic inspiration. The Pumping exercise described above will strengthen the abdominal muscles for the repeated instrokes required for the Cleansing Breath.

Use diaphragmatic breathing, swelling out and drawing in the abdomen, and concentrating on the exhalations, which should be one a second at the start, speeding up to two exhalations a second after three or four weeks' practice. Begin with a round of ten exhalations, and add to this gradually until you are comfortable with twenty to a round. Perform three rounds, with rest pauses between first and second, and second and third, lasting from a few seconds up to a minute, as comfort allows.

Rhythm of performance is important. One tradition gives the durations of inhalation and exhalation as equal, but another tradition says that outbreathing should take only half the time taken by inbreathing. The former is the easier rhythm for beginners; the latter may be acquired later, if you wish.

Dr Behanan (6) says that any of the meditative postures

is good enough as long as *kapalabhati* is practised for a short time, say, four or five minutes. When practised for a longer period, however, the lotus-posture is the only one available. The reason is that when the breathing is carried on over long periods certain vibrations are started all over the body and this, coupled with a feeling of exhilaration, results in a lessening of the motor control over the limbs. But in the lotus-posture the legs are formed into such a firm lock that it is impossible to undo them without the help of the hands, and hence [the legs are] not likely to be disturbed by the lessening motor control.

This shows why the Lotus Posture is considered essential for advanced Yogic practice, but we do not recommend that the home practitioner, using book instruction, should prolong either *Kapalabhati* or *Bhastrika* to the point, mentioned by Dr Behanan, where there is a loss of motor control.

The Cleansing Breath and Bellows Breath are not suitable for persons suffering from high blood pressure, or from eye or ear complaints.

The benefits of the Cleansing Breath are to clear the nasal passages, purify the blood, cleanse the sinuses, remove phlegm, improve circulation, generate *pranic* vitality, tone the nervous system, stimulate the liver, spleen, and pancreas, improve digestion, facilitate evacuation, strengthen and tone the abdominal muscles, and massage the abdominal organs (viscera).

Bellows Breath (Bhastrika)

Bhastrika means 'bellows'. Dr Behanan says (6): '*Bhastrika* is a *pranayama* which is held in high esteem by yogins. This type of breathing is claimed to be best among all the yogic *pranayamas* for arousing the spiritual forces and for preparing the practitioner for concentration (*dharana*) and meditation (*dhyana*).' The Bellows Breath resembles the Cleansing Breath in its first part, and Dr Bernard, when training in Hatha Yoga in India, was taught the former in place of the latter breath control as a purificatory practice. There are several varieties, but all use the rapid bellows-like breathing of *Kapalabhati*. Each version, however, unlike *Kapalabhati*, concludes with a long deep breath, a suspension, and a long slow exhalation – a Complete Yoga Breath, or *Ujjayi* with wide-open glottis.

Version I. This is the most straightforward version, and as efficacious as any. In the first stage, perform the preceding Cleansing Breath ten to twenty times, using both nostrils for inhalations and exhalations. In the second stage, after the final rapid breath, take one slow smooth deep breath through both nostrils, hold it comfortably for a few seconds, and then let it out of the nostrils in a slow smooth continuous flow. This completes one round. The early bellows-like breathing should be vigorous and noisy, though always with rhythmic timing, and the second stage a model of smoothness and control.

Version II. The first stage is as given for version I, but the second stage, like *Ujjayi*, uses a tradition in which one breathes in through the right nostril, keeping the left nostril closed, and then out through the left nostril, keeping the right nostril closed. During retention, both nostrils are closed by the fingers and thumb as will be described and illustrated when we come to the Alternate Nostril Breath. The right hand is not raised at all during the first part of the exercise.

Version III. During the first stage, which is like *Kapalabhati*, inhale and exhale through the right nostril while keeping the left nostril closed. Then immediately take your customary number of rapid breaths (ten to twenty) through the left nostril while keeping the right nostril closed. Follow with *Ujjayi*, using both nostrils and keeping the glottis open.

Version IV. Proceed as in version III, except that you use the traditional *Ujjayi* in which you inhale through the right nostril and exhale through the left nostril, as described for version II.

Version V. Breathe rapidly in and out during the first stage, using only the right nostril. In the slow deep complete breath which follows, again use the right nostril only, keeping the other nostril closed. For the second round use the left nostril only for both stages. For the third round use the right nostril only for both stages. Return to keeping the right nostril closed and the left nostril open for the fourth and final round. Odd numbers – right nostril. Even numbers – left nostril.

Version VI. This is similar to version V; but in the slow final stage breathe in through the nostril which was kept open in the fast early stage, and breathe out through the nostril which was kept closed.

Version VII. During the *Kapalabhati* stage, inhale through the right nostril and exhale through the left nostril during rounds one and three, and breathe in through the left nostril and out through the right nostril during rounds two and four. Procedure in the second stage, the single complete breath, remains the same: inhale through the right nostril and exhale hrough the left nostril.

Version VIII. The first stage is as in version VII, but in the second stage the use of the nostrils corresponds to that in the preceding round of fast breathing. This means that during rounds one and three the *Ujjayi* breath is inhaled through the right nostril and exhaled through the left nostril, but during rounds two and four the roles of the left and right nostrils are reversed.

This by no means completes the number of variations, for some teachers favour the use of the slightly closed glottis during stage one or stage two, or even during both. This produces a sort of sobbing sound in the throat. A somewhat similar effect is produced by the use of the Chin Lock (*Jalandhara Bandha*) during either the *Kapalabhati* or the *Ujjayi* stage, or during both stages.

By first introducing the slightly closed glottis into the eight versions given above; then the Chin Lock; and finally the glottal contraction and Chin Lock in combination, the permutations of *Bhastrika* can be made enormous. Fortunately, I feel we can dispense with both techniques. Slightly closing the glottis serves a purpose in slowing down and introducing a greater element of control into *Ujjayi*, and *Jalandhara Bandha* has its value in advanced *kumbhaka*, but both methods may be omitted without real loss of effect in the Bellows Breath. And as the traditional *Ujjayi* practice of inbreathing with the right nostril and outbreathing with the left nostril is not insisted upon in most modern instruction, our choice of versions to make up four rounds can be made from versions I, III, V, VI, and VIII. In performing four rounds, you can concentrate or combine as you wish, though it is probably desirable that version I should be included at least once.

The benefits are as given for the Cleansing Breath (*Kapalabhati*), though more intense, since a greater intake of air and oxygen results from the complete breath that terminates each round. There are also different physiological effects due to the retention of air between inbreathing and outbreathing during the second stage.

AlternateNostril or Sun and Moon Breath (Anuloma Viloma Pranayama)
Anuloma and *viloma* mean 'with the hair' and 'against the hair' respectively, or, as we might say, 'with the grain' and 'against the grain'.
This is given as a cleansing *pranayama* in the old texts, and makes a gentle alternative for those who find *Kapalabhati* or *Bhastrika* too vigorous. You breathe slowly, smoothly, and deeply through one nostril, the other nostril being held closed, either with the thumb (right nostril) or the ring and little fingers (left nostril) of the right hand. It has the effect of purifying the *nadis* or nerve channels, and its ability to soothe the nervous system and to calm the mind will be apparent from even early practice. This is a most valuable breath control by any criterion.

Before describing the respiratory procedure, it is important to learn the technique traditionally used for closing and releasing the nostrils. No special magical or occult significance need be attached to this particular use of the fingers, but it has been found effective for many centuries.

The index and middle finger of the right hand are folded over and pressed against the palm. The thumb is used to close the right nostril, and the ring and little finger together close the left nostril. Some authorities say that the fingers and thumb should be kept straight; others say that they should be bent at the top joint. Use whichever technique feels most comfortable. To close a nostril,

press against the fatty tissue below the nasal bone so that its inner
surface rests against the septum that divides the nose into two
passages, blocking the nostril on that side. Only gentle pressure
need be applied. Keep your fingernails clear of the tissue (*see*
illustration).

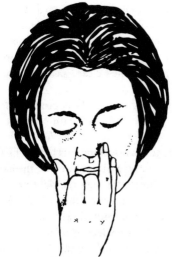

27
**The traditional Yogic method of closing the nostrils during single
nostril breathing**

Left-handed people may, if they wish, use the left hand, closing
the left nostril with the thumb and the right nostril with the ring
finger and little finger of the left hand.

For once the classic texts give straightforward and unambiguous
instruction for practice of this breath control, and are in accord. It
is given as a purification process, prior to the naming and describing
of the main *pranayamas*. A similar type of single-nostril breathing
is included among the main *pranayamas*. This is the Sun Piercing
Breath, so named because the right nostril or 'sun tube' is used
invariably for inhaling.

The *Hatha Yoga Pradipika* gives a straightforward and clear
description of the Alternate Nostril or Sun and Moon Breath (75):

Sitting in the *Padmasana* [Lotus] Posture the Yogi should fill in the
air through the left nostril (closing the right one); and keeping it
confined according to one's ability, it should be expelled slowly through
the right nostril. Then, drawing in the air through the right nostril

slowly, the belly should be filled, and after performing *Kumbhaka* [suspension] as before, it should be expelled slowly through the left nostril. Inhaling thus through the one, through which it was expelled, and having restrained it till possible, it should be exhaled through the other, slowly and not forcibly. If the air be inhaled through the left nostril, it should be expelled again through the other, and filling it through the right nostril, and confining it, should be expelled through the left nostril. By practising in this way, through the right and the left nostrils alternately, the whole of the collection of the *nadis* of the *yamis* [practitioners] becomes clean, i.e. free from impurities, after three months.

The account in the *Siva Samhita* is equally clear (88):

Then let the wise practitioner close with his right thumb the *Pingala* [the right nostril], inspire air through the *Ida* [the left nostril]; and keep air confined – suspend his breathing – as long as he can, and afterwards let him breathe out slowly, and not forcibly, through the right nostril. Again, let him draw breath through the right nostril, and stop breathing as long as his strength permits; then let him expel the air through the left nostril, not forcibly but slowly and gently. . . . He should practise this daily without neglect or idleness.

The account given in the *Gheranda Samhita* is in accord with that given in the other two texts, but adds visualizations (*yantras*) and recitations (*mantras*).

Blow each nostril before practice, and clear it. Some Yogins sniff water and expel it from the mouth after it has appeared in the throat. If one nostril remains partly blocked, it should clear during the exercise. If it is badly blocked, use it for exhaling only for a few rounds.

If one nostril seems more open than the other, this is not surprising, for according to Yoga teaching one nostril predominates in breathing, and the roles are reversed every two hours. During illness this two-hourly rhythm is impaired and one nostril may stay blocked or partly blocked for much longer.

The stages of the Alternate Nostril Breath are as follows:

Sit cross-legged in one of the meditative postures, keeping the head and back erect.

The left hand may be in one of two positions. In the first position, the arm is straightened and the back of the wrist rests on the left knee; in this case it is customary to have the thumb and index finger joined at their tips and to hold the other fingers out straight (*Jnana*

Mudra). Alternatively, let the left hand rest, palm up, in your lap.

Hold the right hand up to the nose, with the thumb and fingers held in the manner described and illustrated above.

Close both eyes.

Close the right nostril by pressing the thumb against the fatty tissue below the nasal bone until it meets the septum that divides the nose into two passages.

Exhale steadily through the left nostril until the lungs feel emptied.

Inhale slowly, smoothly, and deeply through the left nostril, blocking the right nostril, until the lungs feel comfortably filled. Breathe in deeply in the manner already taught, filling the lower, middle, and upper lungs progressively.

Close the left nostril with the ring and little fingers of the right hand. Both nostrils are now blocked.

Hold the breath steadily and easily in the lungs for a few seconds. The Chin Lock may be used, but it is not essential for a short suspension.

Now open the right nostril by lifting the pressure of the thumb against it, but keep the left nostril blocked. Raise the chin from the chest if you have been using the Chin Lock (*Jalandhara Bandha*).

Exhale slowly and smoothly through the right nostril until the lungs feel emptied.

Pause only a second or two before starting inhaling through the right nostril. The left nostril stays blocked. Fill the lungs comfortably.

Close the right nostril with the thumb. Both nostrils are now blocked.

Retain the air for a few seconds without strain.

Open the left nostril by releasing the pressure from the ring and little fingers of the right hand.

Exhale slowly, smoothly, and continuously through the left nostril until the lungs have been emptied.

That completes a round. Perform three to five rounds.

The facial muscles should stay relaxed during the breath control; ideally, the facial expression should be serene.

The traditional texts advise fixing the attention between the eyebrows. The point where the flow of air first strikes the nasal passages is another favoured focusing spot. The aim of such focusing is to steady the mind. Another way of concentrating the mind is to listen to the hissing sound the air makes as it enters and leaves the nose.

The technique of the Alternate Nostril Breath can be briefly summarized as follows:

Having closed the right nostril, effect a preparatory emptying of the lungs through the left nostril before the breath control proper.
Inhale through the left nostril.
Close the left nostril.
Suspend the breath for a few seconds with both nostrils blocked.
Open the right nostril.
Exhale through the right nostril.
Inhale through the right nostril.
Close the right nostril.
Suspend the breath for a few seconds with both nostrils blocked.
Open the left nostril.
Exhale through the left nostril.
Repeat for a second round.

A number of variations are possible. A few rounds may be performed using one nostril for both inhalation and exhalation, without alternating; or you may inhale through one nostril but exhale through both; and so on. But the basic technique is as given in detail above.

Deep and finely-controlled breathing is possible with the Alternate Nostril Breath. The benefits are that it aerates the lungs richly, cleanses the nasal passages and sinuses, purifies the *nadis* or nerve channels, richly oxygenates and purifies the blood, tones and soothes the nervous system, stimulates the appetite, improves digestion, relaxes and refreshes the body, and calms and steadies the mind.

In Sun and Moon breathing the positive and negative *pranic* currents are harmonized and equalized, and the technique of alternate nostril breathing has a role in esoteric Yoga connected with the arousal and control of latent psychic force and the fluctuations and movements of psychic nerve-force within the body.

If for some good reason you cannot perform your full programme of breath controls, then at least perform this one. It can moreover be employed with advantage at times when you particularly need to relax and to calm the mind.

Sun Piercing Breath (Surya Bhedana)
Surya means 'sun' and *bhedana* comes from the root *bhid*, which means 'to pierce'. The sun features in this *pranayama* because you always close the left nostril and inhale through the right or sun nostril, filling the lungs comfortably. You then close the right nostril, so that both nostrils are blocked, and hold the breath for a few seconds, avoiding strain. Open the left nostril by releasing the pressure of the ring and little fingers, and exhale slowly, smoothly, and continuously through the left nostril until the lungs feel emptied.

This completes one round. Perform five to ten rounds. Concentrate the attention as described for the Alternate Nostril Breath.

To summarize the technique:
Close the left nostril.
Breathe in through the right nostril.
Close the right nostril.
Suspend breathing for a few seconds with both nostrils blocked.
Open the left nostril.
Exhale through the left nostril.
Repeat for a second round.

The *Hatha Yoga Pradipika* describes this control succinctly (75): 'Taking any comfortable posture and performing the *asana*, the Yogi should draw in the air slowly, through the right nostril. Then it should be confined within, so that it fills from the nails of the toes to the tips of the hair on the head, and then let out through the left nostril slowly.'

Compare this with the *Gheranda Samhita* (87): 'Inspire with all your strength the external air through the sun-tube [right nostril]: retain this air with the greatest care, performing the *Jalandhara Mudra*. Let the *Kumbhaka* be kept up until the perspiration burst out from the tips of the nails and the roots of the hair.'

Readers without personal supervision should not attempt such prolonged breath-retention, which is common practice under Indian *ashram* conditions. Theos Bernard (7) mentions holding his breath in this *pranayama* for thirty seconds, using the Chin Lock (*Jalandhara Bandha*), and performing ten rounds at the beginning; he worked up to eighty seconds. He was performing *pranayama* four times a day: morning, noon, early evening, and at midnight. This is an old tradition. But he adds that such intensive *pranayama* 'is quite unnecessary for the beginner,' and that 'I was advised never to hold the breath so long that it caused undue strain. It is the repetition of the practice that is recommended, not the use of a great amount of effort.'

Dr Bernard used the Chin Lock (*Jalandhara Bandha*) between inhalation and exhalation, which is customary procedure, but B. K. S. Iyengar (33) in his descriptions of *Surya Bhedana* and Alternate Nostril Breath says that it should be applied prior to the inhalation and that the chin should be kept down throughout the controls.

The benefits are as given for the Alternate Nostril Breath.

Victorious Breath (Ujjayi)

This is another of the main varieties of *pranayama*, and one of the most important. The most widely-practised version uses both nostrils for inhalation and exhalation, and this we will describe first. An older tradition instructs that the breath, after being held, is released through the left nostril. The glottis is partly closed during inhalation and exhalation, producing an audible sound.

Theos Bernard (7) calls *Ujjayi* 'an easy method of deep chest breathing'. That the chest is here expanded is shown by the naming of this *pranayama*, for *jaya* means 'victory', 'triumph', or 'conquest'. The abdomen is kept slightly contracted, and the thoracic cage is expanded fully – a different emphasis from that of the Complete Yoga Breath taught earlier.

Sit in one of the meditative postures, keeping the spine and head erect. As no manipulation of the nostrils is required in this version, the hands stay cupped in the lap, or the arms are straightened so that the back of the left wrist rests on the left knee and the back of the right wrist rests on the right knee, the thumbs and index fingers together and the other fingers held out straight in the gesture known as *Jnana Mudra* or Symbol of Knowledge.

Exhale fully, using either nostrils or mouth. This is preparatory to the start of the Victorious Breath proper.

Draw air in through both nostrils in a slow and continuous flow, whose evenness is measured by its being made audible by partly closing the glottis, the opening from the pharynx into the windpipe which modulates speech and which can be felt to close in swallowing. This partial closure means that the air enters more slowly, and as well as being felt, it is heard to be regulated by the frictional sound produced. The indrawn air strikes the palate with a cool, soft, brushing effect. Continue the inhalation until the lungs feel full, though not so full that they seem about to burst. The prime mover in making this deep inhalation is a full expansion of the thoracic cage. The abdomen is slightly contracted and drawn slightly back to form a flat surface from breastbone to pubic bone. A slight raising of the chest at the end of inspiration helps this. Note how here the action differs from the more diaphragmatic and abdominal emphasis of the Complete Yoga Breath.

Hold the breath comfortably for a few seconds. The glottis is here closed. Dr Bernard was taught to swallow and then use the Chin Lock (*Jalandhara Bandha*). Again B. K. S. Iyengar differs from most accounts in operating the Chin Lock throughout inspiration, suspension, and expiration, and teaches the use of two *bandhas*, *Uddiyana* and *Mula*, during the *kumbhaka*. In the former the abdominal wall is pulled back towards the spine; in the latter the sphincters of the anus are squeezed tightly. But I repeat that the seals need only be used by advanced students.

Now let the air out slowly, smoothly, and continuously through both nostrils until the lungs feel emptied. The glottis having been partly opened, again we hear the regulated sound as the breath flows. Raise the chin from the chest if you have used the Chin Lock.

That completes a round.

Beginners should take exactly the same length of time for inhalation (*puraka*) and for exhalation (*rechaka*), and also for suspension (*kumbhaka*) if comfort allows – a ratio of 1:1:1. For intermediate students the ratio may be 1:1:2 or 1:2:2. Only advanced students should attempt 1:4:2. This means that if five seconds is taken for inhaling, then beginners may suspend breathing for five seconds and exhale for five seconds. Intermediate students inhaling for five seconds may suspend breathing for either five or ten seconds, and exhale for ten seconds. Advanced students inhaling for five seconds may suspend breathing for twenty seconds, and exhale for ten seconds. The unit of time taken in inhaling may gradually be increased with practice.

In summary, the Victorious Breath (*Ujjayi*) is simply described:

Inhale through both nostrils.

Suspend breathing (without raising a hand to the nose).

Exhale through both nostrils.

The above method was taught to Theos Bernard and to Dr Behanan, and is now taught by leading authorities, though the performance of the exhalation (*rechaka*) deviates from what is described in the traditional texts. The *Hatha Yoga Pradipika* gives this description (75):

> Having closed the mouth the air should be drawn again and again through the nostrils in such a way that it goes touching from the throat to the chest, and making noise while passing. It should be restrained, as before, and then let out through *Ida* [the left nostril]. This removes *slesma* [phlegm] in the throat and increases the appetite. . . . *Ujjayi* should be performed in all conditions of life, even while walking or sitting.

The right hand has here to be raised to close the right nostril at the exhaling stage. This version is now little used: students are now told to exhale through both nostrils.

Ujjayi may be practised on occasions while walking or lying down, without using a Chin Lock or any other seal. The benefits are that it invigorates and increases vital capacity, richly oxygenates and purifies the blood, removes phlegm, improves thoracic mobility and broadens the chest, improves digestion, tones the nervous system, and can be used at times when courage is needed.

A traditional therapeutic claim is that it prevents and cures asthma and consumption. According to the *Hatha Yoga Pradipika* (75), 'It destroys the defects of the *nadis*, dropsy and disorders of *Dhatu* [humours].' The *Gheranda Samhita* says (87): 'All works are accomplished by *Ujjayi Kumbhaka*. He [the Yogi] is never attacked by phlegm-disease, or nerve-disease, or indigestion, or dysentery, or consumption, or cough; or fever, or [enlarged] spleen. Let a man perform *Ujjayi* to destroy decay and death.'

Hissing Sound Breath (Sitkari)

This *pranayama* is unusual in that inhalation (though not exhalation) is through the mouth. The lips are slightly parted and the tip of the tongue is thrust between the upper and lower sets of teeth. This means that the tip of the tongue is between the lips; enough space is left between the tongue and the upper lip for air to be drawn in, producing a hissing sound. The air strikes freshly on the forepart of the tongue, and has a cooling effect. When the lungs are comfortably inflated, the lips are closed; the breath is held for a few seconds, and then it is exhaled *through the nostrils*. Perform this three times.

Theos Bernard was taught a different method. He was told to bring the teeth together and to 'float' the tongue in the mouth so as not to touch any part, and then to suck air in between the teeth. With this method too there is a hissing sound, and the effect is cooling. Exhalation, following a suspension, is through the nostrils.

Some aspects of the effects described in the *Hatha Yoga Pradipika* will appeal particularly to male readers (75):

Sitkari is performed by drawing in the air through the mouth, keeping the tongue between the lips. The air thus drawn in should not be expelled through the mouth, but by the nostril. By practising in this way, one becomes next to the God of Love in beauty. He is regarded adorable by the Yoginis [female Yogis] and becomes the author and destroyer of the cycle of creation. He is not afflicted with hunger, thirst, sleep, or lassitude. The *Sattva* of his body becomes free from all the disturbances. In truth, he becomes the lord of the Yogis in this world.

Likewise, surely, the Yogini must become 'next to the Goddess of Love in beauty' and be 'regarded as adorable by the Yogis'.

The benefits are that the Hissing Sound Breath purifies the blood, cools the system, appeases hunger and quenches thirst, and prevents and cures diseases, according to traditional claims.

Cooling Breath (Sitali)

Sitali means 'cool'. *Sitali* is closely related to *Sitkari*, inhalation again taking place through the mouth and exhalation through the nostrils. And again the tongue is pushed between the teeth, but this time the outer edges are curled up to form a trough through which the air is drawn. The tongue is kept between the lips, with the tip protruding slightly beyond them. Draw air slowly and smoothly along the folded tongue. This has been compared to drinking air through a straw.

Then draw the tongue back into the mouth and bring the lips together, holding the breath.

Finally, let the air out smoothly and continuously through both nostrils.

Perform three times.

'This *Sitali Kumbhaka* cures colic, [enlarged] spleen, fever, disorders of bile, hunger, thirst, and counteracts poisons,' says the *Hatha Yoga Pradipika* (75). And the *Gheranda Samhita* says (87): 'Draw in the air through the mouth (with the lips contracted and the tongue thrown out), and fill the stomach slowly. Retain it there for a short time. Then exhale it through both the nostrils. Let the

Yogin always practise this *Sitali Kumbhaka*, giver of bliss; by so doing he will be free from indigestion, phlegm and bilious disorders.'

Theos Bernard was taught the method described above, but he was also given an alternative method in which, during inhalation, the tongue was turned back in the mouth until it was touching the soft palate.

The benefits are that the Cooling Breath purifies the blood, cools the system, quenches thirst, stimulates the liver and spleen, improves digestion, and calms the nervous system and mind.

Bee Breath (Bhramari)

Bhramari means 'bee'. This is sometimes called the Droning Beetle Breath. The ears are closed with the thumbs – the right ear with the right thumb and the left ear with the left thumb – and one listens to the air being drawn into the lungs and squeezed out of them, breathing through both nostrils. The smoothness of breathing can be studied in this *pranayama* by listening to the evenness of the sustained and continuous sound.

The description in the *Hatha Yoga Pradipika* makes a distinction between the sounds of inbreathing and outbreathing (75): '*Bhramari* consists in filling the air with force, which makes a noise like a male bee, and in expelling it slowly which makes a noise like a female bee; this practice causes a sort of ecstasy in the minds of Yogindras.'

The mention of ecstasy shows the connection between this *pranayama* and the concentration (*dharana*) and contemplation (*dhyana*) of Raja Yoga practice. The *Gheranda Samhita* makes it clearly a meditative exercise, concentrating and stilling the mind, and lists many internal sounds to be listened to (87): 'The first sound will be like that of crickets, then that of a flute, then that of a beetle, then that of bells, then those of gongs of bell-metal, trumpets, kettledrums, *mrdanga*, military drums, and *dundubhi*, etc. Thus various sounds are cognised by daily practise of this *Kumbhaka*. Last of all is heard the *Anahata* sound rising from the heart.' These sounds are to be heard, and concentrated upon, during the breath-retention or *kumbhaka*. An 'ah' sound may be uttered low in the throat, causing the palate to vibrate.

Swooning Breath (Murchha)

Here we have mystical experience again. The swooning is by the mind, either during breath retention (the attention being firmly fixed between the eyebrows), or as the breath is slowly released.

The *Gheranda Samhita* says (87): 'Having performed *Kumbhaka* with comfort, let him withdraw the mind from all objects and fix it in the space between the eyebrows. This causes fainting of the mind and gives happiness. For, by thus joining the *Manas* [Mind] with the *Atman* [Soul], the bliss of Yoga is certainly obtained.' And the *Hatha Yoga Pradipika* has this to say (75): 'Closing the passages with *Jalandhara Bandha* firmly at the end of *Puraka* [inhalation], and expelling the air slowly, is called *Murchha*, from its causing the mind to swoon and giving comfort.'

Dr Bernard was taught to sustain a suspension of breathing with the air locked outside the lungs in this *pranayama*, in addition to retention until the mind 'swooned' on filled lungs. He warns (7): 'The beginner is advised not to work on this practice during his preparatory period.'

In *Murchha* the Chin Lock (*Jalandhara Bandha*) is used during retention of breath and during exhalation, though beginners are permitted by their *gurus* to use it only for the former.

Floating Breath (Plavini)
This is a most unusual *pranayama*, for it is practised while floating on water. The legs are crossed – into the Lotus position, each foot upturned on the opposite thigh, if you can manage it – and the head is thrown back. The hands are crossed behind the head to support it. You inhale deeply, suspend breathing, and float easily with a light and buoyant feeling.

It is significant that the posture adopted here is called, when transferred to performance on dry land, the Fish Posture (*Matsyasana*).

The *Hatha Yoga Pradipika* is succinct but poetic (75): 'When the belly is filled with air freely circulating within the body, the body easily floats even in the deepest water, like the leaf of a lotus.'

ADDITIONAL BREATHING EXERCISES

We have now described the main traditional *pranayamas*. The concluding two breathing exercises are simplifications of esoteric 'psychic force' controls.

Pranic *Breath*
This is an exercise in imagination as well as in breath control.
Prana, or cosmic energy, is potently present in oxygen. In this
breathing exercise, which in mechanical performance is straightforward deep breathing – inhalation, retention, exhalation – one
adds visualization and the feeling of rich quantities of *prana* being
taken in on inspiration and then being directed to every part of the
body, feeding blood, nerves, vital organs, tissues, bones, and hairs,
with its life-force.

Prana is the life-enhancing principle pervading the whole
universe, moving the stars in their courses, and operating, in
progressively finer qualities, on physical, mental, and spiritual levels
in Man. Muscular movement is a gross and obvious manifestation,
and thought a subtle manifestation. In Yogic meditation the aim is
to refine thought itself until it reveals its source.

Solar Plexus Charging
This is more localized and concentrated in its effects than the
preceding *Pranic* Breath.

The solar plexus is a complex of nerves at the pit of the stomach,
and is connected with the sympathetic nervous system. It has a
strategic situation in the centre of the body. This is one 'centre' or
chakra whose importance occidentals will recognize: some writers
identify it with the *manipura chakra* of Kundalini Yoga.

Take deep controlled breaths through both nostrils, and through
an act of psychic direction concentrate the drawn-in *prana* in this
storage centre in the pit of the stomach. As you hold your breath
for a few seconds, stockpile *prana* in the region of the solar plexus,
which should become warm.

This is a useful exercise in mind-control, skill in which builds
the ability to warm any part of the body by directing the attention
to it.

Yogic therapy consists of sending *prana* and warmth by conscious
control to damaged or diseased parts of the body, or of directing
healing force to another person's body by laying on hands.

AIMS AND USES OF YOGIC BREATHING

We conclude this section by summarizing the various aims and uses
of Yogic breathing (*pranayama*), not all of which are completely
practical for Western man.

The Daily Programme of Pranayama

Fifteen to twenty minutes should be devoted to *pranayama* each day, selecting exercises from those given above. Of these, *Sitkari* and *Sitali* are somewhat specialized, and most effectively brought into use during hot weather or at times when the practitioner is overheated; this is certainly true of *Plavini*. The basis of a sound effective programme is Cleansing Breath (*Kapalabhati*) or Bellows Breath (*Bhastrika*), or Alternate Nostril Breath if you find these too vigorous. This should be followed by Alternate Nostril Breath and/or Victorious Breath (*Ujjayi*). The other breath controls may be introduced to provide variety, these form the foundation. If you are short of time – though you must have a good reason for not finding it – Alternate Nostril Breath or Victorious Breath (*Ujjayi*) can be practised unobtrusively at some time during the day, the latter while walking if that is the only real opportunity.

The daily session of Yoga breathing increases vital capacity, energizes, exercises the lungs and the respiratory muscles, oxygenates and purifies the bloodstream, removes phlegm, cleanses the sinuses and the *nadis* or nerve channels, soothes and tones the nervous system, improves thorcacic mobility and broadens the chest, improves digestion, massages the abdominal viscera, and calms and concentrates the mind. In addition, the regular programme of *pranayama* brings success in establishing heathful breathing habits, as detailed below.

Establishing Heathful Habits of Breathing

This results from practice of the daily Yogic breathing programme, and from mastering the Complete Yoga Breath given as additional training. These train the thoracic, diaphragmatic, and abdominal muscles to operate efficiently at all times, the habits established in conscious training being carried over into everyday activities, even during the important hours of recuperative sleep.

In the first few weeks of practice the daily programme should be reinforced by making spot checks on your breathing several times a day – while sitting at an office desk, perhaps, or simply reading at home; while travelling to a place of work; or while lying in bed just before going to sleep. At such times play the beam of your attention over the respiratory muscles and make sure they are not being cramped by poor or awkward posture, or by tight clothing, and that your breathing is deep and relaxing, building up the many benefits

to physical and mental health that result from Yogic breathing as a
daily habit, some of which have been listed in the previous section.

Pranayama *at Moments of Need*
There are occasions when one needs to be lifted out of fatigue and
energized, to let go and relax, or to dispel annxiety or fear and to
boost courage. At such times *pranayama* can be brought into use:
Alternate Nostril Breath to relax and vitalize, Victorious Breath
(*Ujjayi*) to energize and give courage. When you are overheated or
during hot weather, *Sitkari* and *Sitali* will cool the system.

Pranayama *for Equanimity and Serenity*
Equanimity has been defined as 'evenness of mind; that calm temper
or mental firmness which is not easily elated or depressed.' Serenity
is 'calmness; quietness; stillness; calmness of mind; evenness of
temper.' To be serene is to be unruffled, like the surface of a quiet
lake mirroring the sky. The Latin *serenus* means 'clear', and serene
has a poetic meaning as a noun – 'the clear expanse of cloudless sky'.
     Spotting the practical significance of the link between the
emotions and breathing was a manifestation of genius on the part
of the sages who first developed *pranayama*. We all know how
excitement and agitation accelerate the rate of breathing; that
nervous breathing is fast, jerky, and shallow; that relaxed breathing
is slow, steady, and deep. But these sages saw the potentialities of
using slow controlled respiration to calm body, mind, and spirit.

Pranayama *as Preparation for the Yoga of Meditation* (*Raja Yoga*)
Slow, deep, quiet breathing conduces to meditative states of consciousness. In some Yogas it is itself a technique for attaining higher
consciousness. And in Buddhist, Taoist, and some other Yogas, the
act of breathing becomes a focus for mindfulness. In Raja Yoga
pranayama may serve to make the breathing so quiet and restful
that it can be forgotten, leaving the attention free for one-pointing
and concentration (*dharana*).
     Patanjali, the author of the key work systematizing Raja Yoga,
treats *pranayama* as one of the eight *angas* or limbs of Yoga, but
devotes very few *sutras* or aphorisms to it. Patanjali knew he could
leave practical instruction in the breath controls to the *gurus*. The
stilling of the mind in his overriding purpose. It is in the classic
texts of Hatha Yoga – the *Hatha Yoga Pradipika*, the *Siva Samhita*,

the *Gheranda Samhita* – that we find more detailed instruction, though even here, as we have seen, the information would be inadequate and confusing were it not for the oral teacher – pupil (*guru – chela*) tradition already in operation when they were written, transmitted down through the centuries to our own day.

Closing the eyes and concentrating on the gentle ebb and flow of breath and the rise and fall of the respiratory muscles induces moods and states of consciousness that are indisputably meditative. In some schools of Yoga *pranayama* is itself a form of meditation.

We know that the achievement and maintenance of health and vitality and the unfolding of higher states of consciousness are both goals found in Yoga, and that some Yogins put the emphasis more on one than the other. But even the Yogin who gives his attention almost entirely to the attainment of glowing health cannot fail to become aware of the reciprocal relationship between respiration and movements within the psyche. Even the most complex and subtle emotions have their concomitant breathing tones, and one discovers that Yogic breathing refines the emotions and the textures and vibrations of consciousness itself. In the highest states of consciousness breathing becomes quiescent and imperceptible. In the folklore of many countries the breath is equated with the soul or spirit. In Genesis 2:7 we find: 'And the Lord God formed man of the dust of the ground, and breathed into his nostrils the breath of life; and man became a living soul.' And in the Gospel According to St John 22:21: 'Jesus *breathed* on his disciples and said, Receive the holy spirit.'

Pranayama *as a Technique in the Yoga of Latent Energies* (*Laya or Kundalini Yoga*)
Pranayama – in particular the *kumbhaka* or breath retention – is applied in its most intensive form in the esoteric Yoga concerned with the awakening and control of vital air or currents (*vayu*) within the body. But long breath suspensions are called for, and this is not a Yoga that can safely be taught by book instruction; personal supervision by a qualified instructor is necessary, and difficult to obtain.

Pranayama *as a Healer: Breathing Therapy*
Yogic breath control may be used as a therapy. Here the principle of *prana* or life-force is much involved. Its flow may be directed by

the practitioner to injured or diseased parts of his own body, or by the laying on of hands or psychic concentration to the body of another.

Pranayama for the Performance of Extraordinary Feats
Levitation, *tumo* (engendering heat), and burial alive are three bizarre and unusual feats that are linked with mastery over breathing. Exhibitions of remarkable powers are, however, frowned upon by responsible Yogins, and public demonstrations of such powers are usually by fakirs and ascetics who have acquired Yogic mastery over body and mind.

The last two uses of *pranayama* listed above will be given separate chapters. But before going on to these, let us take thought for the quality of the air we breathe.

VII Poisonous Air and Vital Air

AIR POLLUTION

Clean dry air is a mixture of gases: 78.9 per cent nitrogen, 20.94 per cent oxygen, and 0.97 per cent other gases. If breath is life, then it is essential that the air we breathe should be fresh, pure, and adequately oxygenated. Water pollution affects mainly the nation causing it, but air contamination may be spread around the world. When a nuclear device is exploded, people thousands of miles away may receive radio-active fall-out. On the brighter side, strong winds help to disperse dirty air.

Great Britain, with her coal-based economy, has had an air pollution problem since Elizabethan times, when wood for burning was becoming scarce. Queen Elizabeth I prohibited the burning of coal in London while Parliament was sitting, but the citizens had no protection most of the year. John Evelyn, the famous diarist, wrote of London during the reign of Charles II: 'Her inhabitants breathe nothing but an impure and thick mist, accompanied with a fulginous and filthy vapour, which renders them obnoxious to a thousand inconveniences, corrupting the lungs, and disordering the entire habit of their bodies; so that Catharrs, Phthisicks, Coughs and Consumptions, rage more in this one City, than in the whole earth besides.' Evelyn did not just fulminate: he put forward sensible remedies. He advised that industries causing smoke should be moved five or six miles out of London, and that trees and shrubs should be planted in the city.

Killer Smog
The situation became much worse in London, and in other smoky British cities, with the Industrial Revolution. From the time of the

Industrial Revolution until comparatively recently, London suffered periodic attacks from killer smog, a combination of smoke and fog, as its name reveals. The term is sometimes used erroneously for chemical and other air-polluting concentrations that do not combine both smoke and fog. Smog occurs when smoke, fog, and low temperatures coincide with a temperature inversion: a layer of cold air becomes trapped under a layer of warm air and gathers smoke and fumes. This situation recurrently causes ill-health and deaths in areas in many parts of the world.

That London is no longer the city of smog is due to action finally taken to combat it in 1956, when the Clean Air Act was implemented. The spur to action was over four thousand deaths in London caused by five days of acute smog in December 1952. Another smog blanket over the metropolis in 1956 caused more than one thousand deaths. Other British cities suffered fatalities from the same cause in 1952 and 1956.

There is another type of smog that may occur during hot weather. During one week in July 1970, this photochemical smog made many thousands of people ill in Buenos Aires, Los Angeles, Milan, New York, and Tokyo.

Industrial Air Pollution
The main air pollutants produced by industry are carbon monoxide, sulphur dioxide and sulphur trioxide, nitrogen oxides, and hydrocarbons. Winds, fortunately, break up and disperse the poisons to some extent, but under certain conditions there can be a build-up of polluted atmosphere in one area to a dangerous degree. Scientists are still struggling to gain an accurate estimate of the possible long-term effects of chemical atmosphere pollution.

Injury to Health
Newspapers, radio, and television report instances of dramatic injury to health and fatalities caused by concentrations of pollutants; but there is also a continuous and gradual damage to health that goes unreported. Elderly people suffer most. Air pollution causes and worsens bronchitis and emphysema. Chronic bronchitis, at the time of writing, is fourth among the major causes of death in Great Britain. The attack on the body by air pollutants takes different forms. Carbon monoxide is preferentially absorbed by the blood. Sulphur dioxide forms an acid solution that eats into lung

tissue – which is also damaged by solid particles. In smoky cities it is rare for doctors carrying out autopsies to see a pink lung; when they do they deduce that the dead person has not been in the city long. Other parts of the body may be damaged; the main effect of photochemical smog is eye irritation.

Governments, somewhat tardily, have been taking action of late, though much remains to be done in many parts of the world. In the USA responsibility remains with individual states, though the Federal Clean Air Act (1963) and the Air Quality Act (1967) mean that the Government can advise and give financial aid to control pollution.

AIR AS FOOD

Yogins hold that air is our most essential food, and that one should seek to breathe air of the highest nutritional value, meaning highly charged with *prana* or life-force. The most vitalizing air, they say, is by the sea, in the mountains, by lakes, and in large open spaces. Modern scientific investigation shows that these areas, which Yogins associate with high concentrations of *prana*, have atmospheres marked by negative ionization. This makes Professor Robert E. Ornstein, a research psychologist at the Langley Porter Neuro-psychiatric Institute in San Francisco, say (115):

The presence of the minutely charged atmospheric ions may constitute a physical analog of the esoteric 'energy form' of *Prana*. In the Hindu tradition, *Prana* is held to be the 'life force', from which health and creativity flow, the force which aids in physical as well as psychological growth. At this point, we cannot measure precisely how much overlap there is between negative air ions and the concept of *Prana*, but some interesting similarities do exist. The esoteric traditions have long taken advantage of favourable microclimatic conditions for their students. Esoteric psychological schools have often been located on mountain tops, near waterfalls, near the ocean. Some recent biological studies have determined that the ionization of the air in these places is predominantly negative.

Many aspects of esoteric tradition stress that when breathing exercises are performed, 'time and place' must be taken into account. The 'time' is the acknowledgement of the rhythmic structure of man. The 'place' may refer, in part, to the presence of the favourable microclimate – negative ionization. The relationship between breathing and consciousness has been little explored by contemporary psychology, but has been stressed in esoteric tradition. As it does for 'body energies', our colloquial language preserves some of the dimensions of this relationship. To note one instance, 'inspiration' refers to both creativity and the process of breathing.

AIR IONS

An ion, *Nuttall's Standard Dictionary* tells us, is 'the electrified particle produced when an atom loses or gains one or more electrons by electrolytic dissociation, or when a molecule of a gas loses an electron through X-ray action.'

In 1899, Elster and Geitel proved that atmospheric electricity depends upon the presence of gaseous ions in the air. Equipment was produced that could indicate the number of ions in the air, and generators were able to produce them. It was found that small air ions are formed when enough energy acts on a gaseous molecule to displace an electron, the latter joining with an adjacent molecule (negative molecular ion), and that the original molecule is positively charged (positive molecular ion).

The number of ions in the air varies from 50 to as much as 10,000 in a cubic centimetre. The number is higher during the day than during the night, higher on unclouded days than on clouded days, higher in summer than in winter. The balance between negative and positive charged ions also varies, depending on several factors. Thunderstorms add to the number of positive ions; so does cloud. Negative charged ions predominate on sunny days, and also on mountaintops. Electricity in the air produces ions, and even the flame from a household fire ionizes. There are large and small ions: the number of large ions increases after sunset, and the number of small ions in the first hours of morning. Investigations show that it is the small ions that have the direct physiological influence, though the large ions have an indirect influence.

Negatively Ionized Air

In a Japanese survey (107), people were asked to give their responses to the atmosphere in rooms with varying quantities of ions and a varying balance between negative and positive ions. When there were few ions the people in the room found the atmosphere 'close'; when positive ions predominated they found the room 'sultry'; 'light and cool' was the response to the introduction of more negative ions, and 'light and fresh' when there was a boost of both negative and positive ions.

The feeling of freshness we experience in the proximity of water-falls and fountains is not just psychological – the air around them is high in negatively charged ions. In Russia, Germany, France, and Italy the ionic content of the atmosphere of spas near waterfalls was studied and found to have a high negative charge. In contrast, positive ions are present in abnormally high amounts in photo-chemical smog, and in those 'winds of ill-repute' (the Mistral, the Khamsin, the Santa Ana, and the Foehn) which raise the incidence of phyiscal and mental ill-health wherever and whenever they blow.

Ions and Air Pollution

Air pollution of the kinds discussed earlier reduce ion levels in the atmosphere: this is found even far out at sea where air pollutants have drifted from the land. Unless we do more to defeat air pollu-tion, mankind faces growing dangers from ion loss as well as from irritation to the lungs and respiratory passages. Professor A. P. Kreuger, a leading investigator of the effects of varying ion levels and balances in the atmosphere, asks (109):

> Will the smogs, hazes and invisible pollutants we generate with a lavish hand so reduce the small-ion content of the atmosphere that plants, animals, and man must suffer harmful consequences? Although the early result of ion depletion very likely will be unimpressive compared to the immediate and dramatic action of known toxic com-ponents of polluted air, this alone should furnish little solace. We have every reason to be aware from past experience that adverse effects may follow continued exposure to a small amount of a minor irritant (e.g. organic solvents) or the long-term deprivation of an essential metabolic requirement (e.g. trace elements or vitamins). The ultimate dimen-sions of biological changes produced by air-ion loss conceivably may prove to be as disenchanting as some revealed by Rachel Carson in *The Silent Spring*.

On the brighter side, Professor Kreuger foresees the eventual regulation of negative-positive air ion balances and levels for com-fort in living and working quarters, just as we already have tempera-ture and humidity regulation. There is a potential use for air ions in stimulating agricultural production. Experiments have shown that the growth of plants is regularly accelerated by high concentrations of either negative or positive air ions (109). And additional negative or positive charges have been found to speed up the germination of silkworm eggs and the growth rate of the developing larvae.

But it is the treatment of disease and the enhancement of health that most interests us here.

Ionization and Health

A. P. Kreuger and others have also studied the effect of positively charged and negatively charged air ions on the breathing of some mammals. They found that a positively charged atmosphere was associated with congestion of the bronchial tubes, a reduced flow of mucus, slow working of the cilia of the windpipe, and a disturbed peristaltic reflex. But when the mammals were exposed to negative ions, the bronchial tubes expanded and relaxed, mucus flowed freely, the cilia of the windpipe worked busily, and peristalsis became normal.

In experiments made at the Institute of Hygiene, Prague, men were exposed to air ions for an hour three times a week for eight weeks. It was found that positive ions induced a rise in blood pressure, a drop in blood albumen, and an increase in the globulin content of the blood; whereas exposure to negative ions raised the blood albumen and lowered the globulin.

A. L. Tchijevsky (118), a Russian scientist, reported to an International Conference on Therapeutic Radiation that 'ion therapy can lead to improvement in eighty-five per cent of patients with vascular and cardiac conditions, hypertension, angina, bronchitis, migraine, endocrine disturbances, allergies, burns, bronchial asthma, and stomach ulcers.'

Other reports indicate that treatment by negative air ions relieves headache, dry mucous membrane, nasal blockage, and irritation of the respiratory tract; and also that negatively charged air produces greater relaxation throughout the whole organism, with an increase of haemoglobin, red blood cells, and iron in the blood. But working out the correct amount of increase of negative ions in treating patients has presented problems. Too strong or too frequent a dose can be harmful – like an overdose of some vitamins. And while some persons are very sensitive to negative ions, others show the opposite characteristic.

Raising and lowering ion levels in the atmosphere of a room, and altering the balance between negative ions and positive ions, are known to influence human moods and states of consciousness. Professor Robert E. Ornstein asks (115): 'Could the introduction of negatively ionized air produce results similar to those achieved by difficult and esoteric breath manipulations?' He refers to the breath controls of Yoga, Sufism, and so on. Insufficient evidence is available so far to give a clear answer to the question, but enough is available to justify the raising of the question.

SMOKING AND HEALTH

While the individual person may not be in a position greatly to influence the cleanliness of the air breathed in our cities, there is one concentrated pollution, the commonest and most dangerous, over which he does have full control – he can choose whether or not to inhale cigarette smoke into his lungs.

The link between heavy cigarette smoking, and lung cancer and some other diseases, is indisputable. The first report of a Committee set up by the Royal College of Physicians of London in 1959 was published in 1962, under the title *Smoking and Health*. The 1962 report said that 'diseases associated with cigarette smoking cause so many deaths that they present the most challenging of all opportunities for preventive medicine.' A second report, *Smoking and Health Now*, published in 1971, says: 'The challenge remains. The total number of deaths attributable to cigarette smoking rises year by year and is likely to do so unless there are radical changes in smoking habits,' and adds, 'the suffering and shortening of life resulting from smoking cigarettes have become increasingly clear as the evidence accumulates. Cigarette smoking is now as important a cause of death as were the great epidemic diseases such as typhoid, cholera, and tuberculosis that affected previous generations.'

The reports of the Committee set up by the Royal College of Physicians of London are unequivocal, and the findings are supported by scientific investigations in several parts of the world. The link between smoking cigarettes and disease and death has been clearly established. But here we are concerned not only with deaths

from lung cancer and diseases caused by the smoking habit, but
with the multiplication of cases – running to millions – of people
who are inflicting upon themselves lower standards of health.

Increased Death-risk for Smokers

The nicotine addict says, along with Charles Lamb:

> For thy sake, Tobacco, I
> Would do any thing but die.

But the risk of dying prematurely is exactly the risk that he
takes, according to the most influential surveys of the hazards
associated with the smoking habit.

The most important of the scientific studies are these: R. Doll
and A. B. Hill, 'Mortality in relation to smoking: ten years' observations of British doctors', *British Medical Journal*, 1964. H. A.
Kahn, 'The Dorn study of smoking and mortality among US
veterans: report of 8½ years of observations', *National Cancer
Institute Monograph*, 1966. E. W. R. Best, 'A Canadian Study of
Smoking and Health', Department of Health and Welfare, Ottawa,
1966. E. C. Hammond, 'Smoking in relation to the death rates of
one million men and women', *National Cancer Institute Monograph*,
1966.

The four investigations came up with similar and unequivocal
findings:

Cigarette smokers have a shorter life-expectancy than non-
smokers.

The greater the number of cigarettes smoked daily, the greater
the death-risk.

Cigar or pipe smoking is less hazardous than cigarette smoking,
but still produces an increased death-risk.

There is a link between cigarette smoking and lung cancer, heart
disease, arterial diseases, chronic bronchitis and emphysema. Some
non-smokers get these diseases, but the risk of having them is much
higher in smokers, especially heavy smokers.

These smoking habits increase the hazards to health and life:
inhaling tobacco smoke; keeping the cigarette between the lips as
you puff; smoking a cigarette down to a tiny stub; and relighting
partly-smoked cigarettes.

These investigations also came up with some encouraging news
for smokers: give up cigarette smoking and you run a steadily
diminishing risk of dying from the effects. Hammond, in his study

of one million men and women, found that when light smokers broke the habit, after ten years their death risk was on a par with non-smokers.

A poster published in Britain by the Health Education Council informs us that:

Every time you inhale from a cigarette tiny particles of nicotine and other chemicals are left inside your lungs. These particles gradually build up into an oily tar that irritates your lungs till they become clogged or infected with phlegm and pus. Then, as more of this septic discharge forms, the mixture of tar, phlegm and pus sometimes rises up into the throat and is swallowed. But the rest of it slithers deep into the lungs, where it congeals and festers. It is not surprising that smokers cough, are short of wind, have bad breath, and are more susceptible to crippling incurable diseases.

Breaking the Smoking Habit

The truth about will-power is that the power comes easily when we really want to give up something. Irritating and fouling the lungs with tobacco smoke is totally opposed to the aims of the practices of Hatha Yoga, which are cleansing and health-enhancing. If he practises Yogic breath controls regularly, the smoker loses the craving for cigarettes and usually cuts down, and then finally drops the habit. A relaxed and healthy system has no need for the stimulation provided by nicotine, and blackening the lungs with inhaled smoke becomes unthinkable.

VIII   Yogic Breathing and Health

THE UNIQUENESS OF *PRANAYAMA*

Dr Kovoor T. Behanan, in his still-pertinent scientific evaluation of Yoga first published in 1937, reported a series of experiments measuring the oxygen consumption in *Kapalabhati, Bhastrika,* and *Ujjayi.* One would expect all three to cause an increase in oxygen consumption over normal breathing and, from he nature of performance, that *Bhastrika* would induce a greater oxygen consumption than *Kapalabhati,* and *Ujjayi* a greater consumption than *Bhastrika.* This, in fact, proved to be the case, the increased consumption over normal breathing for *Kapalabhati, Bhastrika,* and *Ujjayi* being 12.0, 18.5, and 24.5 per cent respectively. It should be remembered that the first two are rapid cleansing breaths, with a different role in *pranayama* from that of *Ujjayi,* which is deep breathing, filling the lungs to comfortable capacity.

That Yogic breathing enhances health and aids healing has been discovered in practice by thousands of people from all walks of life, ranging in age from young to old. Oxygen consumption is increased above that of normal breathing, that much is clear – but so too is it increased by numerous forms of active exercise. Wherein then lies the special merit of *pranayama* ?

Here is Dr Behanan's opinion as to what makes *pranayama* unique as bodily exercise (6):

> Increased oxygen consumption, which is characteristic of yogic breathing, in itself does not mark it off as different from other kinds of exercises, because any kind of exertion involves an increase in metabolic rate which is manifested by the greater intake of oxygen. A few details, like the tipping of the head [Chin Lock] during the holding period and inspiration and expiration with half-closed glottis, may

appear to be unique features. Until we have positive evidence concerning the physiological changes introduced by these details, however, it does not seem reasonable to believe that they are a very important part of the system.

This view remains reasonable almost forty years later. D. Behanan continues:

One thing seems rather unique. In yogic breathing, while the respiratory muscles are exercised in the execution of deep cycles, the other groups of muscles remain relatively inactive. Thus it differs markedly from the deep breathing incident to riding a bicycle. Here, although the trunk and arms are rather inactive, they can hardly be relaxed and the lower limbs are called upon to do vigorous exercise.

The different stages of the respiratory act are executed with calculated deliberation. The contraction and relaxation of the respiratory muscles are accomplished slowly, while jerky movements are avoided. It would seem reasonable, therefore, to believe that *the chief purpose of the yogic breathing exercises is to increase the consumption of oxygen with the minimum of physical exertion, under conditions probably favourable to the storage of oxygen.*

(The italics are mine.)

To this I would add that there are significant differences which elevate *pranayama* above not only other forms of physical exercise that activate deeper breathing, but also the other much less well-known systems of breathing exercises for health (such as the Muller method). These are the basic insistence upon rhythm and smooth control; the retention (*kumbhaka*); and the unique regard for the reciprocal relationship between respiration and the mental state. Search as you may, you will find nothing similar in range and depth of importance to *pranayama*. No other system dares to contemplate Yoga's sublime aim: to perfect body, mind, and spirit.

YOGIC BREATHING AS HEALER

Yogins hold that *prana* is the force behind the renewal of the body cells, and that disease is unlikely to gain a hold on a body whose every body cell is permeated with *pranic* energy. Further, a body freshly charged with *prana* can be a source of healing for others, by transmission. It is especially effective with certain specific complaints.

Asthma and Bronchitis
Deep breathing of the Complete Yoga Breath type is widely
employed in physiotherapy throughout the world. Diaphragmatic
and abdominal breathing relaxes the respiratory muscles and gives
relief and therapeutic benefit in ailments like asthma and bronchitis,
where tension adds to the trouble. Some doctors recommend Yogic
breathing exercises for asthmatics. During asthmatic attacks the
muscles controlling the bronchioles go into a spasm and air gets
into the lungs, but has difficulty in getting out. The sufferer adds
to his problem if he gives way to panic and tries to force air into
lungs already distended. Training in Yogic breathing gives the
asthmatic confidence and the ability to relax and control the
respiratory muscles. The Alternate Nostril Breath and the Victorious Breath (*Ujjayi*) may be practised between attacks with
retention, and during attacks without retention. They may also be
practised by people with bronchitis.

Persons suffering from asthma, bronchitis, and other respiratory
complaints tend to avoid physical exercise, so that their general
health suffers. Yoga practice, with its gentle approach, gives them
exercise, greater confidence, and control.

Colds ,Catarrh, and Sinus Trouble
Yogic breathing prevents head colds and is helpful in clearing up
catarrh and sinus troubles. In particular this is true of the Cleansing
Breath (*Kapalabhati*), the Bellows Breath (*Bhastrika*), and the
Alternate Nostril Breath (*Anuloma Viloma Pranayama*).

Nervous Tension
Nervous tension causes muscular contractions and rigidities in many
parts of the body. As there is a close link between the emotions and
breathing, anxiety, fear, and other stresses result in the respiratory
muscles becoming constricted, so impairing free functioning and
deep breathing.

Neurosis
The value of deep breathing as a therapy for neurotic conditions
was mentioned earlier, when we pointed out that psychotherapists
of the Reichian school use deep-breathing exercises to break up the
rings of muscular tension with which the neutoric 'armours' himself
in the upper body, originally to inhibit emotional expression. Such

self-inflicted strait-jacketing of the respiratory apparatus may persist long after any psychological need for inhibiting emotional expression has passed. In particular, Reich attached importance to his patients learning to exhale thoroughly.

Insomnia
Controlled breathing calms the nervous system and relaxes body and mind. Breathing smoothly and rhythmically on first going to bed keeps away the tension and nervous activity so often responsible for sleeplessness or sleep of poor quality.

Headaches
These are often eased by the Alternate Nostril Breath. The practice of Yogic breathing corrects most of those various conditions that are responsible for headaches.

Indigestion
The practice of *pranayama* improves appetite and aids digestion.

Abnormal Weight
Breathing has an important role in metabolism, the process by which the body uses nutritive elements – which provides a clue to the reason why many people who take up Hatha Yoga find the weight of the body normalizing, the obese losing weight and the thin gaining it. Factors other than respiratory control are likely to be involved, but more efficient breathing is thought to play a part.

Constipation
The abdominal massage given by the Cleansing Breath (*Kapalabhati*) and the Bellows Breath (*Bhastrika*) stimulates natural peristaltic action in the intestines and aids regular elimination of waste matter from the bowels. Performance daily of Abdominal Retraction (*Uddiyana*) and Isolation of the Recti (*Nauli*) is a must for persons who tend to suffer from this complaint.

Compulsive Smoking
An increased and sensitive respect for the body develops with Yoga practice, and blackening and polluting the lungs with inhaled smoke is soon seen as an intolerable affront to bodily hygiene. Yogic

breathing exercises have been found to undermine the craving for nicotine that grips smokers so powerfully, so that the smoking habit loosens its hold and fades away without the smoker being aware of any great struggle of the will.

It can be seen that breathing exercises act as a substitute for smoking: air is inhaled, retained, and exhaled, but it is fresh pure air in place of poisonous air that destroys health. And Yogic breathing, and Yogic practice in general, is more successful than smoking cigarettes in combating restlessness and taut nerves.

HEALING OTHERS

The Yogin who wishes to heal should first build up *prana* in his body and become a channel whereby the cosmic life-force can pass into the patient. Healing is preceded by controlled breathing, charging the body with *prana*, which is usually visualized as being stored in the region of the solar plexus. The healer may also think of *prana* flowing in the *nadis* or nerve channels, and of drawing in the energy of the elements – fire, air, earth, and water.

The Yogin about to heal must be fully rested. The patient is told about the universal life-force, whose healing power he is about to receive. The transmission of energy is usually by the healer placing the palms of his hands flat against the patient's spine and drawing them down it while he (the healer) exhales. This, performed from five to ten times, provides a general vitalization, after which the right hand of the healer is applied to the diseased or damaged part of the patient's body.

After the act of passing *pranic* force to the patient, the healer should lie on his back for some minutes in the Corpse Posture (*Savasana*), resting and recharging.

The most direct link between breath and healing is found in Chinese Taoist breathing therapy. In what they consider the most potent of their treatments, the Taoist healers place cotton wool on the body part affected, and the healer breathes rhythmically on it with parted lips, warming the area.

SELF-HEALING

In Taoist Yoga one comes across methods of self-healing and life prolongation on lines similar to Hatha Yoga's control of bodily

energy currents. The following account (113) of how breath control
and meditation can be combined for self-healing could equally well
be a description of the technique of Hindu Yoga.

The cure for specific maladies is thus described:

> One harmonizes the breath, then swallows it and holds it as long as
> possible; one meditates on the affected part, by thought one pours the
> breath upon it and by thought makes the breath fight the malady by
> attempting to force its way through the obstructed passage. When the
> breath is exhausted, one expels it, then begins again from twenty to
> fifty times; one stops when one sees sweat running over the affected
> part. One repeats the procedure daily at midnight or at the fifth watch,
> until a cure is effected.

A later Chinese text describes the same technique applied in
sequence to all the body's vital organs. As Ssu-ma Ch'eng-cheng
says in his *Discourse:* 'Those who absorb the breaths . . . must
follow them by thought when they enter their viscera, so that the
humours [of the viscera] shall be penetrated [by the breaths], each
[breath] conformably with the [inner organ] over which it presides,
and thus they can circulate through the whole body and cure all
sicknesses.'

LONGEVITY AND YOGA

Exaggerated claims for the longevity of Indian Yogins – that they
live for hundreds, even thousands, of years – do damage to Yoga's
credibility among Westerners, who may on reading this sort of
thing be put off trying techniques, physical and psychological, that
greatly enhance the quality of everyday living. Such statements are
on a par with those that claim that some Yogins can fly like birds
across the Himalayas, or at the very least across a troublesome
gorge or ravine. What *can* be stated with certainty – and impressive
it is – is that some elderly Indian Yogins display a bodily tone and
lissomness and a mental alertness that men half their age in any
country in the world would be delighted to possess.

It is noteworthy that those living creatures that breathe more
slowly tend to live longer than those with rapid breathing rates. A
few comparative figures may be pondered:

A monkey	about 30 breaths a minute
A hen	about 30 breaths a minute
A dog	about 28 breaths a minute
A cat	about 24 breaths a minute
A duck	about 20 breaths a minute
A horse	about 16 breaths a minute
A man	about 15 breaths a minute
A tortoise	about 3 breaths a minute

Some writers on Yoga put forward the theory that as master Yogins breathe more slowly (though more efficiently) than the average citizen, therefore they live longer. A corollary of this argument is that the practice of *pranayama* prolongs life. This is difficult to prove – but it can be safely said that Yogic breathing adds life to one's years, whether or not it adds years to one's life. Probably it does both for many people. Indian Yogins measure their lives, it is said, by the number of breaths they take rather than by minute and hours.

All this leads to puzzling problems as to the nature of chronological, physiological, and psychological time; and intriguing hypotheses arise and are presented.

Professor Eliade, an erudite investigator of Yoga, particularly in its philosophical, metaphysical, and metapsychological aspects, relates a personal experience that illustrates our discussion of a possible link between longevity and the practice of *pranayama*, and a certain link between Yogic breathing and youthfulness (**104**):

I have been struck, at Rishikesh and elsewhere in the Himalayas, by the admirable physical state of the yogins, who took hardly any nourishment. At my *kutiar* at Rishikesh one of my neighbours was a *naga*, a naked ascetic who spent almost the whole night practising *pranayama*, who never ate more than a handful of rice. He had the body of a perfect athlete; he showed no sign of under-nourishment or fatigue. I wondered how it was that he was never hungry. 'I live only by day,' he told me; 'during the night, I reduce the number of my respirations to a tenth.' I am not too sure that I understand what he meant; but may it not simply be that, the vital duration being measured by the number of inhalations and exhalations, which he reduced to a tenth of the normal number during the night, he was living, in 10 hours of our time, only one tenth as long – namely one hour? Reckoning by the number of respirations, the day of 24 solar hours was lived, by him, in no more than 12 to 13 breathing-hours: by the same measure, *he was eating a handful of rice, not every 24 hours, but every 12 or 13 hours*. This is only a hypothesis which I do not insist upon. But so far as I know, no one has yet given a satisfactory explanation of the astonishing *youthfulness* of some yogins.

In the work – *Images and Symbols* – in which this experience is related, Professor Eliade explains how the Yogin advanced in *pranayama* is existing in a different 'time' from that of our ordinary waking consciousness:

Pranayama, by rendering the respiration rhythmic, transforms the yogin, little by little, into a cosmos: breathing is no longer a-rhythmic, thought ceases to be dispersed, the circulation of the psycho-mental forces is no longer anarchic. But, by working thus upon the respiration, the yogin works directly upon the time that he is living. There is no one adept in Yoga who, during these exercises, has not experienced quite another quality of time. In vain have they tried to describe this experience of the time lived during *pranayama*: it has been compared to the moment of bliss that comes when listening to good music, to the rapture of love, to the serenity or plenitude of prayer. What seems certain is that, by gradually slowing down the respiratory rhythm, prolonging the inhalations and exhalations more and more, and leaving as long an interval as possible between these two movements, the yogin lives in a time that is different from ours.

IX   Extraordinary Feats

EXTRAORDINARY FEATS

In this section we will look briefly at three of the most extraordinary feats performed by Yogins – each of which depends for success on advanced skill in *pranayama*. Two of them – burial alive and 'resurrection' many hours later, and *tumo* (engendering body heat) – are fully authenticated; the third feat – levitation – cannot be said to have been performed under conditions that would satisfy the scientifically-minded investigator.

BURIAL ALIVE

In 1926 Harry Houdini, the most famous escapologist, did something almost unknown among magicians – he revealed the secret of one of his most mystifying performances.

In 1974 the Mining Enforcement and Safety Administration in Washington found on their files a letter from Houdini that had been put away and (seemingly) forgotten: it revealed, for the benefit of miners who might find themselves trapped underground with a meagre supply of air, the technique Houdini used to survive $1\frac{1}{2}$ hours in a sealed iron coffin at the bottom of the swimming pool of New York's Shelton Hotel. The letter was written four months before Houdini died. 'I know you are doing worthwhile work,' he wrote, 'and as my body and brain are trained for this particular line I am at your service.' He went on to tell how, struggling with heat nausea, hallucinations, and the urge to sleep, he controlled and conserved his breathing so as to live for ninety-one minutes on an air supply that would normally suffice for only five minutes of life.

Houdini, as with the method of swallowing and regurgitating a key mentioned in the chapter on the cleansing processes, had again hit upon a Yogic method of bodily mastery. However, the technique of burial and 'resurrection' displayed on many occasions by Yogins in India is more radical and prolonged than Houdini's, and involves going into a trance state. The performer needs to have full trust in the associates who bury him and who massage him 'back to life'. There have been some fatalities.

Major F. Yeats-Brown, who served for twenty years in the Bengal Lancers, gave one description of burial alive in the *Sunday Express*, London:

Resurrection of the 'dead' is a fairly common exercise in Indian magic. I have seen it done twice. The adept undergoes twenty-four hours of secret preparation, which consists in purgation, fasting, and 'swallowing' air.

Before the trance state is induced, the adept is in a state of oxygen intoxication. Then, pressing his carotid arteries, he passes into unconsciousness.

His disciples bury him.

On one of the occasions when I was present, the adept remained thus for an hour, on the other occasion he remained in the death-trance for only fifteen minutes.

Doctors who examined the 'corpse' stated that there was no sign of life. When the given time had elapsed, the adept came to life.

It is not an experiment fit for public view, the rigid body un-stiffens, the set lips relax, and from them issues a groan that none who have heard it can forget.

In February 1936 the *Sunday Times*, Madras, reported that a Yogi named Swami Vidyalankar, in the presence of several doctors, had reduced his heartbeat to unrecordable levels. 'He also showed several other feats, including that of remaining buried in a pit for 25 hours.'

In the same year, *The Madras Mail* reported:

BURIED ALIVE FOR THIRTY MINUTES
Yogi's feat witnessed by 15,000 people

Masulipatam, Dec. 15.

A remarkable feat of Yoga was exhibited by Yogi Sankara Marayanaswami of Mysore on Sunday evening in front of Sri Ramalingeswaraswami's Temple in the presence of a gathering of about 15,000 people. He was buried alive for about half an hour.

Lt.-Col. K. V. Ramana Rao, I.M.S., District Medical Officer, who acted as observer, took a letter from the Yogi before the ordeal, stating that he was performing the feat on his own responsibility.

The Yogi was seated in a box specially prepared for the purpose and let down into a pit, which was covered with earth. After about half an hour, the box was removed, when the Yogi was found sitting in a state of trance. The Yogi regained consciousness half an hour afterwards, when he was cheered by the people.

The most detailed description of the feat comes from the pen of a German doctor (106):

Runjeet Sing was told that a *saat*, or faqueer, living in the mountains, was able to keep himself in a state resembling death, and would allow himself to be even buried, without injuring or endangering his life, provided they would remove or release him from the grave after the expiration of a fixed time, he being in the possession of the means of resuscitating himself again. The maharajah thought it impossible. To convince himself of the truth of the assertion, he ordered the faqueer to be brought to court, and caused him to undergo the experiment, assuring him that no precaution should be omitted to discover whether it was a deception. In consequence, the faqueer, in the presence of the court, placed himself in a complete state of asphyxia, having all the appearance of death.

In that state he was wrapped in the linen on which he was sitting, the seal of Runjeet Sing was stamped thereon, and it was placed in a chest, on which the maharajah put a strong lock. The chest was buried in a garden, outside of the city, belonging to the minister, barley was sown on the ground, and the space enclosed with a wall and surrounded by sentinels. On the fortieth day, which was the time fixed for his exhumation, a great number of the authorities of the durbar, with General Ventura, and several Englishmen from the vicinity, one of them a medical man, went to the enclosure. The chest was brought up and opened, and the faqueer was found in the same position as they had left him, cold and stiff. A friend of mine told me, that had I been present when they endeavoured to bring him to life, by applying warmth to the head, injecting air into his ears and mouth, and rubbing the whole of his body to promote circulation, etc., I should certainly not have had the slightest doubt of the reality of the performance. The minister, Rajah Dhyan Sing, assured me, that he himself kept this faqueer (whose name was Haridas) four months under the ground, when he was at Jummoo in the mountains. On the day of his burial, he ordered his beard to be shaved, and at his exhumation his chin was as smooth as on the day of his interment; thus furnishing a complete proof of the powers of vitality having been suspended during that period. He likewise caused himself to be interred at Jesrota, in the mountains, and at Umritsir, and also by the English in Hindostan. In the *Calcutta Medical Journal* about 1835, there is a full description of the faqueer, and we are there informed that he preferred having the chest in which he was enclosed, suspended in the air, instead of its being buried beneath the earth, as he feared the possibility of his body being attacked by ants whilst in that middle state between life and death.

The German doctor was interested in Haridas's preparation for burial, which included some of the purification practices of Hatha Yoga.

Doubtless it is a difficult task, and not within the power of everyone, to acquire the skill necessary for the performance of this experiment, and those who do succeed must undergo a long and continual practice of preparatory measures. I was informed that such people have their *froenulum linguoe* cut and entirely loosened, and that they get their tongues prominent, drawing and lengthening them by means of rubbing with butter mixed with some pellitory of Spain, in order that they may be able to lay back the tongue at the time they are about to stop respiration, so as to cover the orifice of the hinder part of the *fosses nasales*, and thus (with other means for the same purpose, which I shall mention) keep the air shut up in the body and head. Novices, in trying the experiment, shut their eyes, and press them with their fingers, as also the cavities of the ears and nostrils, because the natural warmth of the body might cause such an expansion of the enclosed gas as otherwise to produce, by the violence of its pressure, a rupture of some of those delicate organs not yet accustomed by practice to endure it. This, I am told, is especially the case with the eyes and the tympan of the ear. For the better acquisition of this power, they are accustomed to practise the holding of the breath for a long period.

They swallow a small strip of linen, in order to cleanse the stomach, and by a tube draw a quantity of water through the anus into the intestines to rinse them. This is performed while sitting is a vessel filled with water to the height of the arm-pits. It is said that the faqueer in question, a few days previous to his experiments, took some kind of purgative, and subsisted for several days on a coarse milk regimen. On the day of his burial, instead of food, he slowly swallowed, in the presence of the assembly, a rag of three fingers in breadth and thirty yards in length, and afterwards extracted it, for the purpose of removing all foreign matters from the stomach. . . .

These preparations being made, the faqueer stopped all the natural openings in the body with plugs of aromatic wax, placed back his tongue in the manner I have before indicated, crossed his arms over his breast, and thus suffocated himself, in the presence of a multitude of spectators.

On his exhumation, one of the first operations is to draw his tongue into its natural position; after this, a warm aromatic paste, made from pulse meal, is placed on his head, and air is injected into his lungs and also through the ears, from which the plugs are withdrawn. By this operation, the pellets in the nostrils are driven out with considerable force and noise, and this is considered the first symptom of his resuscitation. Friction is then strenuously applied all over the body, and at length he begins to breathe naturally, opens his eyes, and is gradually restored to consciousness.

TUMO

Tumo is the technique of engendering body heat at will. Here again we have a control of importance to persons struggling for survival – this time in conditions of severe cold.

A detailed account of *tumo* is given by the French traveller and writer Mme Alexandra David-Neel, who visited remote parts of Asia. In her book *With Mystics and Magicians in Tibet* (103) she calls *tumo* 'the art of warming oneself without fire up in the snows'. This art enables hermit Yogins to spend the winter in snow-girt caves at altitudes between 11,000 and 18,000 feet, wearing only a single thin cotton garment, or even no clothing at all.

Tumo means 'heat' or 'warmth', but with various levels of meaning, from the gross bodily heat that can melt snow to 'fires' within the subtle body.

Tibetan adepts of the secret lore distinguish various kinds of *tumo*: exoteric *tumo*, which arises spontaneously in the course of peculiar raptures and, gradually, folds the mystic in the 'soft, warm mantle of the gods'; esoteric *tumo*, that keeps the hermits comfortable on the snowy hills; mystic *tumo*, which can only claim a distant and quite figurative connection with the term 'warmth', for it is the experience of 'paradisiac bliss' in this world.

In the secret teaching, *tumo* is also the subtle fire which warms the generative fluid and drives the energy in it, till it runs all over the body along the tiny channels of the *tsas*.

The *tsas* – the nerves, veins, or arteries of the subtle body – correspond to the *nadis* of Hindu Yoga, and the technique of kindling 'subtle fire' corresponds to the Hatha Yogin's awakening of serpent power (*kundalini*).

Mme David-Neel adds: 'However, only a few, even in mystic circles, are thoroughly acquainted with these several kinds of *tumo*, while the wonderful effects of the *tumo* that warms and keeps alive the hermits in the snowy wilds are known to every Tibetan.'

Initial cleansing breaths and later breath retentions are an essential part of the method, but these are combined with techniques of concentrative meditation, in which mystic syllables and fire are visualized vividly. In one method the sun is imagined in the palm of each hand, below the navel, and on the sole of each foot. The suns in the hands and in the feet are rubbed together, kindling the sun below the navel, which blazes up and fills the whole body with fire.

By combining advanced breath controls with intensive use of concentration and imagination, naked or skimpily-clad Yogins, sitting cross-legged and immobile, meditate for hours on exposed mountain slopes in sub-zero temperatures. Much as a Western Boy Scout is given some task whereby he gains an extra badge, so the Tibetan neophyte is given a test to prove his ability in engendering body heat. The test is to sit wrapped in a sheet that has been dipped in icy lake water. Dry three of these wet sheets in succession with your body heat, and you qualify for the title 'Respa', or Cotton-clad One. Qualified monks have been known to cheat and wear other clothing below their cotton shirt.

A 'little *tumo*' is within the capacities of most 'householder Yogins', and does not require the holding of the breath for several minutes or baroque visualization. With practice in concentrating the mind upon one part of the body, that part can be made to feel warm; and the technique can be extended eventually to the whole body. There are times in life when such adroit use of the powers of attention and imagination can prevent a chill or more serious illness, or simply hasten the onset of refreshing sleep.

LEVITATION

Under the headline 'Sitting in Air' the *Asiatic Monthly Journal* for March 1829 reported an event in Madras (100):

A Brahmin, old and slightly made, represented to be of high caste, contrives to poise himself in a most remarkable manner in the air. He performs this feat at any gentleman's house, not for money, but as an act of courtesy. The following is a description from an eye-witness, given in a Calcutta paper: 'The only apparatus seen is a piece of plank, which, with four pegs, he forms into a kind of long stool; upon this, in a little brass saucer or socket, he places, in a perpendicular position, a hollow bamboo, over which he puts a kind of crutch, like that of a walking crutch, covering that with a piece of common hide: these materials he carries with him in a little bag, which is shown to those who see the exhibition. The servants of the houses hold a blanket before him, and when it is withdrawn, he is discovered poised in the air, about four feet from the ground, in a sitting attitude, the outer edge of one hand merely touching the crutch, the fingers of that hand deliberately counting beads; the other hand and arm held up in an erect posture. The blanket was then held up before him, and they heard a gurgling noise like that occasioned by wind escaping from a bladder or tube, and when the screen was withdrawn he was again standing on terra firma. The same man has the power of staying under water for several hours. He declines to explain how he does it, merely saying he has been long accustomed to do so.' The length of time for which he can remain in his aerial station is considerable. The person who gave the above account says that he remained in the air for twelve minutes; but before the Governor of Madras he continued on his baseless seat for forty minutes.

This is fascinating: but it has all the elements – apparatus 'he carries with him', a blanket held before him – and atmosphere that one associates with a performance by a stage magician. The 'gurgling noise like that occasioned by wind escaping from a bladder or tube' is intriguing – had the old Brahmin, by some practice of *pranayama*, filled himself with air? Certainly this was a performance with which an exponent of the art could make a good living on the cabaret circuits today.

The evidence for levitation is based on only a handful of reports. With all respect to the author of a popular work on Yogic breathing who says that hundreds of Christian saints performed the feat, what evidence there is for levitation (though none of it was taken under conditions that would satisfy a scientific investigator) comes either from India or from Tibet. We will ignore the material of best-sellers that is clearly fiction. But Mme Alexandra David-Neel claims to have seen people levitating in Tibet, and Dr Alexander Cannon claims that he was taught to float through the air over a gorge in the Himalayas (101).

He gave us instructions as to how we should cross this gulf by practising the levitation and transportation formula in which we had become ere this adept in its perfect manipulation.

Within a few hours we made our bodily state fit to allow of this great miraculous transportation phenomenon taking place by pure mental effort, and in another moment of time landed safely on the other side.

Princess Choki of Sikkim, in her description of her uncle's daily levitation (quoted by Fosco Maraini in his *Secret Tibet*), makes the astonishing feat sound as homely as performing press-ups before breakfast. Her last sentence is priceless (111):

He [my uncle] was the most extraordinary man I ever met. I remember that when I was a little girl he . . . did what you would call exercises in levitation. I used to take him a little rice. He would be motionless in mid-air. Every day he rose a little higher. In the end he rose so high that I found it difficult to hand the rice up to him. I was a little girl, and had to stand on tiptoe. . . . There are certain things you don't forget.

To these eye-witness accounts may be added a few lines by Professor Ernest Wood, though it is not clear whether he was actually among the spectators who made a close inspection of an old Yogin who was 'mystically inclined' (91):

Levitation, or the rising of the body from the ground and its sus-pension a few feet up in the air above the seat or couch, is a universally accepted fact in India. I remember one occasion when an old yogi was levitated in a recumbent posture about six feet above the ground in an open field, for about half an hour, while the visitors were permitted to pass sticks to and fro in the space between.

Readers will form their own opinions on the basis of this evidence. Sceptics point out that no religion or ideology is without its mavericks, so it is surprising that not one exhibitionistic yogi has been found who is willing to levitate before scientists or to succumb to the temptation to demonstrate this most astounding of feats in the West or before film cameras – for fame and fortune surely await the first yogi to do so.

What does seem probable is that levitation is often confused with the floating feeling and the sensation of lightness which results from prolonged practice of *pranayama*, and which may be accompanied by hallucinations and the feeling of having become airborne. In his book *The Occult Training of the Hindus* (120), Ernest Wood writes: 'When I tried the long breathing, as a boy of fourteen or fifteen, for three quarters of an hour, I found when I stood up that I had lost my sense of touch and weight. I handled things without feeling them, and walked without any sense of touching the ground.' There are also bizarre accounts of yogins who, having swallowed huge quantities of air, bounce along the ground on their bottoms. The *Siva Samhita* describes it (88): 'Through the strength of constant practice, the Yogi obtains *Bhucharisiddhi* locomotory power , he moves as the frog jumps over the ground, when frightened away by the clapping of hands.' The Tibetan Yogins developed this Tantric technique to amazing lengths, according to the report by Mme David-Neel (103):

The student sits cross-legged on a large and thick cushion. He inhales slowly and for a long time, just as if he wanted to fill his body with air. Then holding his breath, he jumps up with legs crossed, without using his hands and falls back on his cushion, still remaining in the same position. He repeats that exercise a number of times during each period of practice. Some lamas succeed in jumping very high in that way. Some women train themselves in the same manner.

As one can easily believe, the object of this exercise is not acrobatic jumping. According to Tibetans, the body of those who drill themselves for years by that method become exceedingly light; nearly without weight. These men, they say, are able to sit on an ear of barley without bending its stalk or to stand on the top of a heap of grain without displacing any of it. In fact the aim is levitation.

A curious test has been devised. . . . A pit is dug in the ground, its depth being equal to the height of the candidate. Over the pit is built a kind of cupola whose height from the ground level to its highest point again equals that of the candidate. A small aperture is left at the top of the cupola. Now between the man seated cross-legged at the bottom of the pit and that opening, the distance is twice the height of his body. For instance, if the man's height is 5 feet 5 inches, the top hole will be at 10 feet 10 inches from the pit's bottom.

The test consists in jumping cross-legged, as during the training exercises which I have described, and coming out through the small opening at the top of the cupola.

Mme David-Neel says she did not witness this feat herself, but heard from Tibetans that it had been performed. The sitting jumps described above are part of the training of the Tibetan *lung-gom-pas* runners, who are said to run across mountainous country for several successive days and nights without stopping. 'Under the collective term of *lung-gom* Tibetans include a large number of practices which combine mental concentration with various breathing gymnastics and aim at different results either spiritual or physical,' says Mme David-Neel (103).

All the extraordinary feats described in this chapter are possible only, if at all, following years of very advanced breathing practices, well outside the furthest limits of our practical approach to the Yoga of Vitality. And this could be said too of the intensity of breath control taught in the Tantric texts to which we have frequently referred. This is how the *Hatha Yoga Pradipika* describes the stages of *pranayama* (75): 'In the beginning there is perspiration, in the middle stage there is quivering, and in the last or third stage one obtains steadiness; and then the breath should be made steady or motionless. The perspiration exuding from exertion of practice should be rubbed into the body (and not wiped) i.e. by so doing the body becomes strong and light.'

Total dedication of this kind is intended for practitioners being taught *pranayama* by a *guru*. Readers should have a realistic picture of the determination he is likely to be called upon to sustain. 'I experienced the first stage at the very onset,' Dr Bernard (7) recorded.

After one or two rounds the perspiration began to flow freely. As I developed strength and power, it was slower in making its appearance and was not so extreme as when I was straining. It was several weeks before I observed the second stage, quivering, and this was at a time when I was perfecting *bhastrika*. First there appeared itching sensations. As I continued the practice, the sensations increased. Soon I began to feel as though bugs were crawling over my body. While I was working, my leg would suddenly shake. Later, other muscles unexpectedly contracted, and soon my whole body would shake beyond control. At this time I was told always to use the *padmasana* [Lotus] posture. This prevented the body from going into convulsions.

By adhering to my schedule, these manifestations all passed away. Another trying experience resulted from the agonizing pains that pierced the abdominal cavity. At first there were loud croaking noises as the intestines became filled with air. This was caused by swallowing the air as it tried to find its way out. The increased pressure was the source of this problem; but I was told that it would cease in time, and it did. At such periods, if one does not have an understanding of the principles upon which the practices are based, his faith is likely to forsake him. It is difficult to hold in mind the advice of the [*Siva Samhita*] text: 'Verily there are many hard and almost unsurmountable obstacles in Yoga, yet the Yogi should go on with his practice at all hazards; even were his life to come to the throat.'

To quote the *Siva Samhita* again (88): 'In the first stage of *pranayama*, the body of the Yogi begins to perspire. When it perspires he should rub it well, otherwise the body of the Yogi loses its *Dhatu* [humours]. In the second stage there takes place the trembling of the body; in the third, the jumping about like a frog; and when the practice becomes greater, the adept walks in the air.'

X   Yoga and Sexual Health

YOGA AND SEXUAL FITNESS

The physiological factors which enhance sexual fitness are vitality, rich reserves of energy, good muscle tone, supple limbs and joints, and efficient functioning of the nervous system, circulation, and glands. On the psychological side, sexual well-being depends on freedom from tensions and anxieties, a relaxed openness of response, and total attention. Yoga practice promotes all of these factors.

That the disciplines of body and mind required for reaching the heights of contemplation and mystical illumination under the conditions of *ashram* schooling should demand chastity is understandable. There is no question here of repressing a force thought inimical to life, but rather of conservation of powerful life-currents and their transmutation into the finest vibrations of psychic energy. But celibacy (*brahmacharya*) is not asked of the 'householder Yogin' – the family man practising Yoga at home. Instead, it is expected of him that he will utilize sexual union to intensify and heighten his spiritual life. Coitus between loving partners can become an act of Yogic contemplation, taking on some of the qualities of the sacred rite that it becomes in Tantric Yoga. It is frequently reported that the sexual life of husband and wife takes on a fresh vitality and glow, and attains a heightened quality when one partner practises Yoga – better still if both do. The majority of readers of this manual will not wish to adopt chastity, unless for short periods, and will welcome enhancement of sexual health and experience within Yoga's harmonious life-style, based on the perfecting and balancing of physiological, psychological, and spiritual energies.

POSTURES AND SEXUAL VIGOUR

The *asanas* in general, by increasing vitality and lissomness, improve sexual fitness, but specific postures are held to act as restoratives of lost sexual vigour. Among these are the Thunderbolt Posture and the Supine Thunderbolt (in which one lies flat on the back after sitting on the heels in the basic pose), the Shoulderstand, the Plough, the Cobra, the Bow, the Locust, and the Spinal Twist. These, in their various ways, heighten libido, stimulate and tone the sex glands and reproductive organs, improve suppleness and pelvic and spinal mobility, and are beneficial for premature ejaculation, menstrual and menopausal disorders, enlarged prostate, frigidity, and impotence.

But it is certain *bandhas* and *mudras* of esoteric latent-power Yoga that act most directly upon the sexual muscles and organs.

BANDHAS AND MUDRAS

A *bandha* is a 'binding' or 'restraint', and a *mudra* is a 'seal' or 'lock'. Both are techniques for locking the breath and *prana* (or life-force) within the body, and the distinction between them is theoretical. These muscular locks and controls have on the whole been kept secret because of their links with the awakening of psychic powers and the harnessing of sexual energies, and they have been surrounded by unnecessary mumbo-jumbo. They have attracted people interested in occult and magical powers, and aroused prurient interest because they have been so persistently written about in guarded and abstruse language. Passages relating to them in the Tantric texts have been omitted in English translations or translated circumspectly into Latin, thus drawing attention to what the translators wished to conceal – like the old-fashioned bathing costumes.

THE TEN CHIEF MUDRAS AND BANDHAS

The *Hatha Yoga Pradipika* lists ten *mudras* and *bandhas* which 'should be kept secret by every means, as one keeps one's box of jewellery.' They are: *Maha Mudra, Maha Bandha, Maha Vedha,*

Khecari Mudra, Uddiyana Bandha, Mula Bandha, Jalandhara Bandha, Viparita Karani Bandha, Vajroli Mudra, and *Shakti Calana Mudra*. The *Siva Samhita* lists the same ten, but the *Gheranda Samhita* lists twenty-five.

Maha Mudra (Great Sealing)

The left leg is folded and the left heel brought in to press against the perineum (between anus and genitals). The right leg is fully extended, and you bend forward to grasp the toes of the right foot. The Chin Lock (*Jalandhara Bandha*) is applied, lowering the point of the chin into the jugular notch between the collar bones. The anus is contracted, repeatedly and strongly, and the abdomen is drawn back. Breathe deeply, filling the thoracic cavity, and press *prana* (life-force) down. Another life-current, called *upana*, which belongs to the abdominal region, is pushed up, and the two energy currents are united at the navel.

Reverse the roles of the legs frequently in practice. The big toe rather than all the toes may be grasped, or the hands may be locked around the ball of the foot. Beginners may grasp the ankle instead of the foot.

Maha Bandha (Great Binding)

This posture differs from the preceding *Maha Mudra* mainly in the placing of the legs. One heel is again drawn in against the perineum, but the other leg, instead of being stretched out straight, is folded and the foot is placed high up on top of the opposite thigh. Again, it is customary to retract the abdominal wall and repeatedly to contract the anus. And again, the esoteric aim is to unite upper and lower energy currents.

Maha Vedha (Great Piercing)

The sitting position for *Maha Bandha* may be adopted here, or any of the meditative cross-legged postures. A deep breath is taken and then held, the Chin Lock (*Jalandhara Bandha*) being applied. The palm of the right hand is placed on the ground beside the right buttock and the left palm on the ground beside the left buttock. The Yogi then presses down with his hands and bounces gently with his buttocks on the ground a few times. The anal sphincters and the lower abdomen are contracted as if in an attempt to bring anus and navel together. Hold the breath as long as is comfortable;

then release it slowly, at the same time relaxing the muscular contractions.

The *Gheranda Samhita* waxes lyrical (87): 'As the beauty and charms of women are in vain without men, so are *Mulabandha* and *Mahabandha* without *Mahavedha*. . . . The Yogin who daily practises *Mahabandha* and *Mulabandha*, accompanied with *Mahavedha*, is the best of Yogins. For him there is no fear of death, and decay does not approach. This *Vedha* should be kept carefully secret by the Yogins.'

Khecari Mudra
This is not recommended. Each day the frenum or membrane which joins the tongue to the lower part of the mouth is cut a little, until the tongue can be curled back into the gullet to block off the passage of air from the nostrils into the windpipe. In addition, the tongue is pulled out and lengthened by a milking action with the hands, until the tip of the tongue can touch the eyebrows. The intrepid Theos Bernard (7) gives a cut-by-cut account in his 'report of a personal experience'.

An ornate mythology surrounds the esoteric practice of this *mudra*, but it need not concern us here.

Uddiyana Bandha (Abdominal Retraction)
This is retraction of the relaxed abdominal wall on a full exhalation. It is considered to be one of the cleansing processes of Yoga hygiene, as well as a 'binding' in Yogic breath control. Its value as an exercise is what interests us most in our practical approach, and a whole chapter has been given to it and its accompanying muscle control, *Nauli*. Its practice is held by Yogins to improve sexual health.

Mula Bandha
For this exercise it is customary to sit in the Perfect Posture (*Siddhasana*), with one heel against the perineum and the other heel against the pubis. Sit in the Easy Posture if the Perfect Posture is too difficult. Dr Bernard (7) was instructed 'to take a position on elbows and knees'.

Mula means 'root'. The perineum, the soft part between anus and genitals, is contracted. At the same time the sphincters controlling the opening and closing of the anus are tightly squeezed, and so are the genital muscles. The lower abdomen, below the navel, is pulled back towards the spine. Try to pull anus and navel together. Hold the contraction for as many seconds as you can without discomfort. Contract the lower abdomen and whole pelvic area five times, relaxing for fifteen seconds each time between contractions.

Asvini Mudra

Tightening and holding shut the circular anal sphincters, as performed in *Mula Bandha* and other controls, is called *Asvini* or Horse *Mudra*. The contraction is named after the staling of a horse. This is an important muscle control in relation to sexual health and fitness, because the fibres of the anus join with those of the genital area.

Jalandhara Bandha (Chin Lock)

This is the Chin Lock employed to assist in suspension of breathing (*kumbhaka*) in advanced Yogic breath control. The chin is lowered into the jugular notch between the collar bones high up on the breastbone. During breath retention it is often combined with two other 'seals' – *Uddiyana Bandha* and *Mula Bandha*.

Viparita Karani Bandha (Inverted Body Binding)

Though a posture, this is listed in the classic texts among the *mudras*. Theos Bernard gives it as identical with the Headstand Posture (*Sirsasana*), but Ernest Wood describes the Shoulderstand Posture (*Sarvangasana*). The main Tantric texts appear to be describing the Headstand. 'Place the head on the ground and the feet up into the sky, for a second only the first day, and increase this time daily,' says the *Hatha Yoga Pradipika*. 'Place the head on the ground, with hands spread, raise the legs up, and thus remain steady,' is the instruction of the *Gheranda Samhita*. 'Putting the head on the ground, let him stretch out his legs upwards, moving them round and round,' says the *Siva Samhita*.

Vajroli Mudra

This *mudra* is often omitted from translations and discussions of Tantric texts, or is referred to in such guarded tones that dispro-portionate curiosity is aroused. It should be remembered that Trantrism is the Yoga of Sex, and contains a number of occult and magical concepts and practices. These are not the most appealing or practical of Yogic techniques, but the modern reader is entitled to read the texts without resort to Latin. The *Hatha Yoga Pradipika* says (75):

> Even one who lives a wayward life without observing any rules of Yoga, but performs *Vajroli*, deserves success and is a Yogi. Two things are necessary for this, and these are difficult to get for the ordinary people – (1) milk and (2) a woman behaving, as desired. By practising to draw in the *Bindu* (semen) discharged during cohabitation, whether one be a man or a woman, one obtains success in the practice of *Vajroli*. By means of a pipe, one should blow air slowly into the passage in the male organ. By practice, the discharged *Bindu* is drawn up. One can draw back and preserve one's own discharged *Bindu*. The Yogi who can protect his *Bindu* thus, overcomes death; because death comes by discharging *Bindu*, and life is prolonged by its preservation. By preserving *Bindu*, the body of the Yogi emits a pleasing smell. There is no fear of death so long as the *Bindu* is well established in the body. The *Bindu* of men is under the control of the mind, and life is dependent on the *Bindu*. Hence, mind and *Bindu* should be protected by all means.

Here we perceive a concept which has received as yet no scientific backing, but which persists in folk-lore, and in occult, magical, and 'higher knowledge' cults: namely, that retaining semen is a way of conserving life-force. The association of semen with strength, potency, creative power, and the masculine principle in the universe is understandable. As the source of procreation, it was inevitable that it should be credited with magical and occult powers.

The sexual control (not recommended here) of absorbing the ejaculate seems incredible, but one recalls the technique of taking a cup of water into the bladder through the urethra, mentioned in the chapter on Yoga's cleansing processes. The same method is clearly involved here. It is unlikely to 'catch on' as a method of birth control – but what a puzzle for some theologians if it did!

The description of *Vajroli* given in the *Gheranda Samhita* bears no relation to the above sexual control, and is obviously a posture (87): 'Place the two palms on the ground, raise the legs in the air upward, the head not touching the earth. This awakens the *Sakti*, causes long life, and is called *Vajroli* by the sages.'

Shakti Calana Mudra
This is concerned with the arousal of latent psychic nerve-force in the body – symbolically a coiled serpent (*kundalini*) that sleeps

between the rectum and the base of the spine. The symbolism of its arousal and ascent through the vital centres (*chakras*) to the crown of the head is colourful and complex, and belongs to the Yoga of Meditation. Shakti is the female power or principle in nature.

Sahajoli and *Amaroli Mudras*

Two more *mudras* may be briefly mentioned before moving on to the adaptation of some of the preceding muscle controls to enhancing sexual health. They are described along with *Vajroli* in the *Hatha Yoga Pradipika* (75): '*Sahajoli* and *Amaroli* are only the different kinds of *Vajroli*. Ashes from burnt up cow dung should be mixed with water. Being free from exercise of *Vajroli*, man and woman seated at ease, should both rub it on their bodies. This is called *Sahajoli* . . . the *Amaroli* is the drinking of the cool mid stream.'

YOGA AND SEX CONTROL

The prevalent problem of premature ejaculation (the Kinsey inquiry revealed that a majority of American males have an orgasm within two minutes of union) can be countered in several ways, one of which is breath control. Orgasm is triggered off by mounting physiological excitement – pulse rate, blood pressure, and breathing all accelerate during foreplay, eventually bringing about a climax and ejaculation in the male.

Yogins who have developed mind-body mastery to a high degree have control over all three excitatory responses, but for the majority of men it will be the last of the three named, breathing, which lends itself most readily to control. Respiratory regulation is at the centre of the practice of the Yoga of Vitality. Yoga makes use of the calming effect of slow smooth breathing on the total organism. The man who has a rushed orgasm within seconds of entry should learn to stay still and to breathe quietly. There are other supporting methods he can employ – choice of the least stimulating coital position, for example – but the second most important technique is another which Yoga practice induces: an ability to let go, relax the body muscles, and calm the mind's agitation. At the first sign of undue excitement heralding the onset of an orgasm, the man should let go with his body muscles, at the same time relaxing his mind – which may mean visualizing a pastoral scene, or some such act of imagination. Eastern couples sustain coitus longer than Western couples: Western attitudes of hurry, worry, and grab-what-pleasure-you-can-quickly are contributing factors.

For women, the problem is mostly one of not achieving orgasm at all. Here again, relaxation of breathing, musculature, and mind keeps away the kind of psycho-physical tension that militates against sexual fulfilment. Teachers of Hatha Yoga to women report that their pupils frequently report a happier and more relaxed sex life after a few months' regular Yoga practice.

Abdominal Retraction (Uddiyana Bandha)

This has been given a chapter to itself. Among the many benefits of this muscle control is its influence on sexual health and vitality. Besides massaging the abdominal viscera, it tones up the muscles of the pelvic floor, relieves congestion and activates circulation in that area.

Contraction of the Penile Muscles of Erection

The male sexual organ, in responding to sexual excitement, engorges with blood, lifts and rises to an angle above horizontal. The erector penis muscles responsible for the rise and the *transversus pevinei* and ejaculatory muscles contract to press on the root of the penis to 'bind' it and keep blood in the spongy tissues of the organ. Normally, the erection of the penis does not come under conscious control – but the penile muscles of erection can be contracted, toned, and strengthened, whether the penis is flaccid or erect. The result is a short quick 'jerk' that is more visible in an erect phallus. Make ten contractions without pause. Relax a few seconds; then repeat. Relax again for a short time, and repeat.

Contraction of the Penile Muscles of Ejaculation

The ejaculatory muscles can be exercised and brought under conscious control in the following way. When urinating, cut off the flow abruptly by conscious command, releasing the stream of urine again after a cessation lasting five seconds. This should be done several times until the bladder has been emptied.

Contraction of the Pelvic Floor

Both men and women can practise this *mudra*, which benefits sexual health. Hold each contraction strongly six seconds. Five successive contractions is sufficient at any one time. As a result of contracting the pelvic floor, an increased flow of blood circulates in the area, the pelvic muscles are strengthened and toned, and neuromuscular control is sharpened.

We are not born with this control, but we acquire it in training to choose our own times for emptying bladder and bowels. The contraction operates when an adult has to cope with a natural urge to urinate or defecate at a time when circumstances force delay in answering the call. It will be found that contraction of either set of muscles means contraction of both. There is an anatomical reason for this: the fibres of the two sets of muscles intermingle. It is possible to develop control of each set of muscles separately, but our concern here is to contract the whole area from pubis to rectum. Squeeze and draw in the muscles as though you were trying to make navel and anus meet. The more powerful of the two sets of muscles are those of the anus (the anal sphincters). So by directing your command to the stronger anal muscles you normally ensure effective control of the whole area. Later, control of specific parts of the pelvic floor may be acquired.

Contraction of the Vaginal Muscles

These muscles are contracted when a woman urgently wants to empty her bladder but is forced to wait, and in the spasmodic contractions of orgasm. The *bulbo-spongiosus*, which acts as a vaginal sphincter, can be squeezed in, but the opening to the vagina, unlike that to the rectum, is always slightly open, and the muscles usually grip less strongly. A woman can also squeeze in the levator muscle in the wider part of the vagina. Like the rectum, the vagina has two main muscles controlling its action – a sphincter muscle that grips or opens and a levator muscle that draws up. The anal sphincter is trained to grip and open in childhood; the vaginal sphincter tends to be neglected.

In contracting the pelvic floor, the vaginal muscles share in the squeezing in and drawing up. If a woman concentrates her attention upon the sensations experienced in this area, she can develop the grip and pull, influencing sexual health and fitness and increasing the enjoyment of coitus for both partners.

Each contraction should be strongly sustained for six seconds, and ten contractions should be made, with brief relaxation between them. Do not dissipate energy by contracting muscles other than those in the pelvis. After one month's practice, an attempt should be made to contract the vagina separately from the anus. As there is an intermingling of the fibres of the two sets of muscles, separate control will not be one hundred per cent successful, but the relative strengths of the contractions felt in the two parts can be reversed, so that the vaginal squeezing in and drawing up becomes the stronger. At first the vaginal opening (sphincter) will noticeably be felt to contract, but later the sensations in the inner walls will also be experienced and recorded, to act as feedback information for full vaginal muscular control. The acme of this intimate female control is to contract the muscles of the deeper walls separately from those of the entrance. Some women can contract the clitoris separately.

The effects of applying this control during coitus are considerable. i. There are bunches of sensitive pleasure nerves concentrated at the vaginal orifice, which are stimulated by squeezing in the vaginal sphincter. ii. The clitoris, the most pleasurably sensitive of all the female sexual organs, is drawn down towards the phallus. iii. The male's pleasure is also enhanced – so much so, that for a man with the problem of hasty ejaculation it is prudent to leave his partner's 'milking' action until the final rush to climax. The Hindu love-manual, the *Ananga-Ranga*, says: 'To this end, i.e., to give pleasure to the husband, she [the wife] must ever strive to close and constrict the *Yoni* [vagina] until it holds the *Linga* [penis], as with a finger, opening and shutting at her pleasure, and finally acting as the hand of the Gopi-girl, who milks the cow.' iv. The penis can be held in the vagina following ejaculation and during detumescence, adding to the 'afterglow' for both partners, and also lessening the frustrating effects of premature ejaculation, should it occur. If the root of the penis is gripped firmly, blood will drain from the spongy tissues in a slow trickle. v. Where there are potency problems, full erection being difficult to maintain, this female art of vaginal control ensures that the penis is held in the vagina and squeezed repeatedly, assisting firmness. vi. By control of the vaginal sphincter, a woman can retain seminal fluid when she is seeking conception. vii. Lastly, the vaginal contractions tone muscles that may slacken through childbirth or age.

This intimate Yogic muscle control improves a woman's sexual health and well-being. She feels secure in her womanhood and in the knowledge that her sexual efficiency can be maintained late into life.

SEX AND MATURITY

For a fuller account of the use of exercises and muscle controls to improve and maintain sex fitness through the middle years and later, see the author's book *Techniques of Sex Fitness* (Universal, New York). The eminent British sexologist, Dr Robert Chartham, reviewing this work for *Forum*, called it 'one of the most important books on sex and health which has appeared in recent years'. Yogic postures, *bandhas* and *mudras*, provided the basic exercises described in *Techniques of Sex Fitness*, and more briefly in this chapter. It must be pointed out that the increased sexual health and sexual enjoyment that results from these controls will take its place easily and unobtrusively within Yoga's total life-style, which is one of moderation in all things and, when fully developed, of universal love. Of the type of person represented by the perfected Yogin, Alan Watts has written (119): 'for them an erotic relationship with the external world operates between that world and every single nerve ending. Their whole organism – physical, psychological and spiritual – is an erogenous zone. Their flow of love is not channelled as exclusively in the genital system as is most other people's.'

But even those of us who have just taken the first clumsy steps on the path to Yogic perfection will find that the *quality* of our sex life, as well as its vitality, is enhanced by Yogic exercises and controls. And the quality grows with the passing of the years. As I said in *Techniques of Sex Fitness* (105): 'Many men and women find supreme joys in lovemaking late in life when the opportunity presents itself for a kind of distilled sensuality, a blending of fleshly passion and spiritual love with subtle overtones and harmonies denied to clamorous youth. For many men and women the best, sexually, is yet to be.'

TANTRISM

A surviving Indian tradition, of ancient origin, aims at utilizing sexual energy to awaken higher consciousness. There are two contrasting approaches.

In the first approach, sexual energy is conserved through chastity. This is a matter of sublimation, not of viewing sex as sinful or inimical to the spiritual life. The sexual energies are

precious and to be harnessed for self-realization. Yoga increases
sexual energy, but also develops the ability to transmute this energy
into creative mental activity if desired.

However, the student, unless studying with a *guru* under
restricted conditions, is not expected to forego sex. On the contrary, he is encouraged to use yoga to improve the quality and
depth of his love life. Not only are levels of sexual energy raised,
but sexual efficiency is improved in the ways already indicated in
this chapter. Teachers of Yoga in the West say that their pupils
often report an enhancement of the sexual side of their marriages
after a short period of yoga practice.

The second yogic approach to sex makes coitus a sacramental act
of contemplation. The mystical end-goal of yoga is a union of
positive and negative, male and female, *yang* and *yin* forces in the
cosmos. The union of individual Self (*Atman*) and universal Over-
self (*Brahman*) is symbolized in the physical coupling of man and
woman. Much mystical language has sexual connotations – words
like 'union', 'marriage', 'merge', 'dissolve', 'melt', 'bliss', and
'ecstasy'.

Ritual coitus may be actual or a vivid working of the imagination.
Orgasm may be withheld, or permitted after prolonged union,
perhaps for an hour or even two hours.

This second approach – coitus as sacrament – belongs to the
Tantric tradition, which is the subject of my book *Yoga and Meditation*. Among the yogas, Tantrism is unique in character and tone.
It views life as a dance, a play of universal energy, and sees in the
physical union of man and woman a mystical 'way', a path to
transcendental ecstasy.

XI Yogic Diet

CLASSIC GUIDELINES

The dietary instructions of the classic texts are more direct than
those given for the postures and breath controls, but for the
twentieth century occidental they provide guidelines rather than
detailed advice on planning meals, since a high proportion of the
foods listed are difficult to obtain outside of Asia. Nevertheless, it is
worth looking at what the three main source-books have to say.

The *Hatha Yoga Pradipika* (75) lists:

Foods injurious to a Yogi; Bitter, sour, saltish, hot, green vegetables,
fermented, oily, mixed with til seed, rape seed, intoxicating liquors,
fish, meat, curds, *chhaasa* pulses, plums, oil cake, asafoetida [*hingu*],
garlic, onion, etc. should not be eaten. Food heated again, dry, having
too much salt, sour, minor grains, and vegetables that cause burning
sensation, should not be eaten. . . .

Wheat, rice, barley, *sastika* [a kind of rice], good corns, milk, ghee,
sugar, butter, sugar candy, honey, dried ginger, *Parwal* [a vegetable],
the five vegetables, *moong*, pure water, these are very beneficial to
those who practise Yoga. A Yogi should eat tonics [things giving
strength], well sweetened, greasy [made with ghee], milk, butter, etc.,
which may increase humours of the body, according to his desires.

The *Gheranda Samhita* (87) tells us that:

He who practises Yoga without moderation of diet, incurs various
diseases, and obtains no success. A Yogin should eat rice, barley
[bread], or wheaten bread. He may eat Mudga beans [*Phaseolus
mungo*], Masa beans [*Phaseolus radiatus*], gram, etc. These should be
clean, white, and free from chaff. A Yogin may eat *patola* [a kind of
cucumber], jack-fruit, *manakacu* [*Arum Colocasia*], *kakkola* [a kind of
berry], the jujube, the bonduc nut [*Bonducella guilandine*], cucumber,

plantain, fig; the unripe plantain, the small plantain, the plantain stem and roots, *brinjal*, and medicinal roots and fruits (e.g. *rhhi*, etc.). He may eat ghee, fresh vegetables, black vegetables, the leaves of *patola*, and *Vastuka*, the *hima-locika*. These are the five *sakas* (vegetable leaves) praised as fit food for Yogins. Pure, sweet and cooling food should be eaten to fill half the stomach; eating thus sweet juices with pleasure, and leaving the other half of the stomach empty is called moderation in diet. Half the stomach should be filled with food, one quarter with water; and one quarter should be kept empty for practising *pranayama*.

And the *Siva Samhita* (88) says:

Now I will tell you the means by which success in Yoga is quickly obtained . . . The great Yogi should observe always the following observances: – He should use 1. clarified butter; 2. milk; 3. sweet food; and 4. betel without lime; 5. camphor; 6. kind words; 7. pleasant monastery or retired cell, having a small door; 8. hear discourses on truth; and 9. always discharge his household duties with *Vairagya* (without attachment); 10. sing the name of Visnu; 11. and hear sweet music; 12. patience; 13. constancy; 14. forgiveness; 15. austerities; 16. purifications; 17. modesty; 18. devotion; and 19. service of the *Guru*.

From the above three quotations, the general principles of the Yogic approach to diet can be discerned. Note the association in the third quotation of diet and morality. Yogins have reverence for all life, and follow a lacto-vegetarian diet. Westerners who join Indian *ashrams* are expected to adhere to this principle, though Indian *gurus* teaching in the West recommend it but do not insist upon it. And Yogins hold that kinds of food influence consciousness itself.

FOODS AND HUMAN CONSCIOUSNESS

Traditionally, three kinds of food are held to influence human personality: *sattvic* or pure food, *rajasic* or stimulating food, and *tamasic* or impure food. Examples of *sattvic* food are milk, butter, fruit, vegetables, and grains. Examples of *rajasic* foods are spicy and strong-tasting foods, meat, fish, eggs, and alcohol – all of which stimulate the nervous system. *Tamasic* foods are putrefied, overripe, rotten, or impure in some way. Each of these three classes of food has a corresponding state of consciousness: gross, intermediate, and spiritual for *tamasic*, *rajasic*, and *sattvic* foods respectively.

A physician called Charok, attached to the Court of King Kanich Ka, composed a work about 200 AD called *Charaa Samita*, in which he advised on the right diet for health, strength, and longevity. He classified the foods into two main groups: heavy and light (by qualities not weight), corresponding to the above-mentioned *rajasic* and *sattvic* groupings. Heavy foods have the properties of earth and moon, and light foods those of air and heat. The light (or *sattvic*) foods should predominate in a healthful diet. Examples are vegetables, fruit, grains, milk, butter, and cheese.

Yogins say that a growing liking for pure, wholesome, nourishing food is part of a student's spiritual unfoldment, and that progress in Yoga and purity of diet go together.

ALKÁLINE-FORMING FOODS

Most of the *sattvic* foods are alkaline-forming. Health depends on a slightly alkaline pH for the bloodstream. Invading bacteria that could be harmful find themselves in an unfavourable medium. Professor E. V. McCollum, of Johns Hopkins University, says that the daily diet needs a considerable amount of alkaline-forming foods: salads, vegetables, fruits; and a moderate quantity of acid-forming foods: starches, sugars, meat, poultry, fish, eggs, and cheese. The majority of the inhabitants of Western countries eat too many acid-forming foods, causing acidosis, whose symptoms are lassitude, headaches, nausea, insomnia, and loss of appetite.

THE CASE FOR LACTO-VEGETARIANISM

Most Indian Yogins are lacto-vegetarians: that is, they do not eat flesh, but do include milk and milk products in their diet. (The phrase must be 'most Indian Yogins' because some Tantric Yogins eat meat.) They are vegetarians principally on ethical grounds – the association between the purity of the foods we eat and our spiritual development mentioned above, and the cruelty and crudity of killing for food. They also share, with vegetarians throughout the world, doubts about the long-term effects on health of eating meat and meat products.

For thousands of years vegetarianism has been practised by millions of people in the East, where Brahmanism, Buddhism, Jainism, and Zoroastrianism have long held all life to be sacred. Notable people in the West who have been vegetarians (the word was not coined until 1840) include Pythagoras, Plato, Socrates, Ovid, Hippocrates, Seneca, Plutarch, Tertullian, Clement of Alexandria, Leonardo da Vinci, Rousseau, Voltaire, Milton, Oliver Goldsmith, Sir Isaac Newton, Shelley, George Bernard Shaw, Albert Einstein, and Albert Schweitzer.

It is true that millions of people go without meat from circumstances rather than choice: a vegetarian does so on principle. Two groups of vegetarians may be distinguished:

i. Vegans, whose diet consists of fruit, vegetables, nuts, and grains, and who exclude all foods of animal origin, including milk and milk products, and even honey. Nor do they wear clothing obtained by animal slaughter. They follow, as best they can, the idea expressed in Pope's line: 'No murder clothes him, and no murder fed.'

ii. Lacto-vegetarians include milk and dairy products in the diet.

The austere Vegan diet needs very careful planning if it is to provide all essential nutrients, minerals, and vitamins. Advice is given by vegetarian societies found in many countries. The lacto-vegetarian diet has proved itself healthful for millions. Some winning Olympic athletes have been vegetarians.

Vegetarianism, as a chosen life-style, is marked by Yogi-like simplicity, moderation, and spirituality. It may be argued that idealistic and spiritual people choose vegetarianism, rather than that abstaining from flesh makes them the kind of persons they are – but the belief is strong among vegetarians that killing animals and eating them coarsens and harms the psyche, and that only a suspension of imagination prevents the majority of Westerners from giving up killing for food.

Vegetarians believe that, in addition to its being morally degrading, flesh-eating is harmful to health; that the vegetarian diet, if thoughtfully planned, is the healthier of the two. They point out that cancer, degenerative diseases of the heart, and other 'diseases of civilization' are most prevalent in flesh-eating communities; that the anatomy of man is that of a frugivore rather than a carnivore (long bowels, the ferment ptyalin in his saliva for predigesting starches, well-developed salivary glands, incisor teeth, and so on); that the muscle fibres of meat contain large concentrations of uric acid, which the meat-eater has to eliminate, putting a strain on the liver and kidneys; that meat quickly putrefies, releasing poisonous substances, whereas vegetables, fruit, and milk products decay or ferment.

There is a sense, deep down, biologically, in which we are all vegetarians. As David Le Vay (110) writes (the first italics are mine):

The essential chemical elements of protoplasm are carbon, hydrogen, nitrogen, sulphur, and phosphorus. Simple compounds of these, such as water and carbon dioxide, require an elaborate synthesis for their conversion into organic or living matter; this is effected by green plants under the influence of sunlight. Neither man nor animals can achieve this synthesis for themselves; they are dependent on the consumption of vegetable matter, either directly or indirectly, after it has been utilized by other animals lower in the food chain which serve as food in their turn. *Ultimately, we are all vegetarians, and all flesh is grass.* Thus, the energy transformations of living matter begin with light absorbed by plants and end with the heat waste of both plants and animals. In its passage this energy is subject to the laws of thermodynamics and can be utilized to do *work*.

MODERN YOGA DIET

Westerners are well established in their dietary ways, but the student of Yoga should aim to change his diet *gradually* in the ways that follow – if Yogic belief is correct, the more deeply the practitioner goes into Yoga the more he (or she) will be drawn effortlessly to do so.

i. Cut down on meat and meat products. Too much protein is acid-forming. Textured vegetable protein (TVP) from soya and other pulses and grains is now available. Its flavour resembles that of meat and it costs much less. Nuts are a leading source of protein for vegetarians and a substitute for meat. They supply the important B-group vitamins and calcium, potassium, phosphorus, and magnesium. Eventually, some readers may find they wish to give up flesh-eating entirely.

ii. Avoid, as far as is possible, denatured and chemicalized foods, such as white bread, white sugar, and white rice; artificially

sweetened foods; heavily sugared drinks; highly spiced foods; and
highly salted foods.

iii.   Eat a lot of alkaline-forming (*sattvic*) fruit and vegetables.
Swami Vishnudevananda, an Indian teaching Hatha Yoga in
America, says (89):

> the valuable organic mineral elements of iron, potassium, lime, soda,
> etc., which serve as eliminators, antiseptics, blood purifiers, and
> producers of electromagnetic energy are mostly found in the plant
> kingdom. The main supply of organic minerals comes from fruits and
> vegetables. Fruits and vegetables also aid in keeping an alkaline reserve
> in the blood. This is essential in maintaining its capacity for carrying
> carbon dioxide to the lungs for elimination.

He says also that 'fruits and raw vegetables contain antiscorbutic
substances that prevent various diseases.'

iv.   Include milk and dairy products in your daily diet. They
provide materials for growth and repair. Milk's lactic acid bacteria
aid digestive processes. Cheese provides first-class protein, and is a
rich source of calcium. To quote Swami Vishnudevananda again
(89): 'Milk is a complete protein food. Thus, a diet containing milk
and dairy products, fresh fruits, oranges, lemons, and pineapples,
leafy vegetables (salads), and whole grains should be man's ideal
vitamin-rich diet.' In short, a lacto-vegetarian diet.

v.   Make sure you eat some uncooked foods every day. The
British Vegetarian Society recommends that fifty per cent of food
eaten daily should be uncooked. The reason for this is that cooking
destroys vitamins and enzymes, which play a leading role in all life
processes. Temperatures well below boiling point – between fifty-
six and eighty degrees centigrade – destroy many enzymes. Many
processed and tinned foods are deficient in them. The more raw
vegetables that are included in salads the better for health. Add
flavour with herbs. Including more uncooked vegetables, fruits, and
grains in your diet ensures an adequate supply of enzymes and
healthy working of those already in the body.

vi.   Eat some wholewheat bread and uncooked wholewheat each
day. The roughage of wholewheat bread encourages the movement
of food in the intestines and colon, and the bread is rich in B-
complex vitamins and in the minerals potassium, magnesium,
phosphorus, calcium, and iron. There is great satisfaction, and
great benefit to health, in baking wholewheat bread for oneself at

home. Two recipes follow, one using yeast and the other without
yeast.

> A. 1 lb. wholemeal flour
> Just over ½ pint water (blood heat)
> 1 teaspoonful salt
> 1 teaspoonful sugar (or crude black molasses)
> ½ oz. fresh yeast

Warm the flour and mix in the salt. Mix the yeast and sugar with
¼ pt. hand hot water and leave ten minutes to froth up. Stir yeast
mixture and remainder of water into flour and knead dough for ten
minutes. Shape dough into a buttered or floured tin, cover with a
cloth and leave in a warm place for about half an hour (until dough
doubles, to just below top of tin). Bake 35-40 minutes in a moderate
oven.

> B. 1 lb. wholemeal flour
> ¾ pint buttermilk
> 1 teaspoonful bicarbonate of soda
> 1 teaspoonful cream of tartar

Mix a little of the buttermilk with the bicarbonate of soda and
the cream of tartar to form a smooth paste. Mix all the ingredients
together to form a moist dough. Line a tin with a sprinkling of
flour and coat the dough with flour to prevent burning and sticking. Bake for one hour in a moderate oven.

Some readers will recognize this second recipe as the 'wheaten
bread' much enjoyed in Ireland.

Baking the bread should be an act of mindfulness, of total
attention, of Karma Yoga. Kahil Gibran put it beautifully in *The
Prophet*: 'For if you bake bread with indifference, you bake bread
that feeds but half man's hunger.'

Uncooked wheat is superior even to wholewheat bread for
supplying enzymes and vitamin B which, because it benefits the
nerves and digestion, is called 'the happiness vitamin'. It is also a
rich source of vitamin E, which has associations with sexual health.
Purchase organically-grown wheat grains from a healthfood store,
and grind them, using an electric coffee-grinder. Either make a
porridge with the freshly-ground wheat or mix it with water or milk
and leave it covered overnight. In the morning add some of the
following: raisins or chopped dates, nuts, apples, bananas, lemon
juice, honey or maple syrup. This breakfast supplies energy for
several hours and satisfies hunger.

vii.   Keep meals simple. This means having a few foods instead of many at one meal. Include a high proportion of natural fresh uncooked foods.

viii.   Eat moderately. The physician Charok said: 'One should take a proper measure of food.' This means leaving the table feeling one might have eaten a little more – so following the injunction of the classic text quoted earlier to leave a quarter of the stomach empty. As the aims of Yogic training are health, purification, and self-realization, the Yogin's diet should become a part of Yogic practice. This means simplicity and moderation – but never inadequacy. There are Hindu ascetics who seek to ingratiate themselves with the Divine Source by going without food until they are skin and bones. Hatha Yoga texts make it clear that this is not a true Yoga path. The founder of the Buddhist religion tried it and found it a hindrance rather than a help in finding man's essential nature.

ix.   Chew well. The first process of digestion takes place in the mouth, with the mixing of food and saliva. Strong chewing brings maximum flavour out of the food, as well as aiding digestion. Thorough mastication is yet another yoga exercise, and so to be performed with full attention.

CONCLUSION

If the reader has not been content merely to read through this book but has already put its techniques and exercises into practice, then he or she will probably have joined the many people who practise Yoga regularly and who have discovered that such practice improves the quality of living. It does this by improving health and by increasing vitality – and, integrated with the preceding two benefits, by inducing psycho-physical poise and relaxation. This writer first began to study and to experiment with Indian Yoga and Eastern systems of meditation twenty-five years ago at a time when he was writing his first book – on the subject of relaxation. He still feels that relaxation of a profound quality is the greatest benefit that Yoga offers to its European and American practitioners.

The pace and pressures of living in Western technological society destroy health and happiness through what are known as the 'stress diseases' and tensions within the psyche. Doctors estimate that over one million people in Britain suffer from tension headaches – a different problem from migraine, though often mistaken for it. The main cause of the headache is tension in the muscles at the back of the neck. Doctors know only one treatment – to prescribe tranquil-lizing drugs to dull the impact of stress and to reduce the pain. How much better to counter stress with the body's own defences! It is here primarily that Yoga has proved so effective and so valuable for Western men and women.

Posture Programmes For Life

The Yogic postures, by repeatedly stretching the trunk and limbs and because of their serene immobility, smooth away tension in those muscles where it most frequently lodges – in the lower back and in the neck.

The third chapter of this book should establish the reader in the practice of a sound and well-balanced programme of postures. How-ever, after some months there is likely to develop a wish to extend the range of practice. In *Yoga Postures* this writer has described more than four hundred postures, including limber-up exercises and Western adaptations and modifications of classic *asanas*. Books by the Indian masters, however valuable for the serious student, fail to allow for the lack of suppleness of the average European and Ameri-can taking up Yoga. But this reference guide – the most complete ever published – meets the needs of students at every level of strength and suppleness, and there is guidance for planning pro-grammes for beginners, intermediate, and advanced students.

Meditation For Physical Health and Psychological Well-being

Yoga and Meditation – the third volume in a trilogy on Yoga practice – covers a subject touched on only indirectly in the first two volumes. Consciousness is influenced to some extent by the breath controls and postures – but for the deepest changes, bringing serenity and inner freedom, you will need to practise Yoga meditation.

Persons interested in Eastern mysticism and metaphysics will not need any persuading to take an interest in the practice of Yoga meditation. But not all enthusiasts for the 'physical' type of Yoga are attracted by the mental disciplines. However, this indifference or aversion is mostly due to outdated notions of the nature and effects of meditation.

Yoga meditation is a technique, and not a religion. It was devised thousands of years ago to silence the 'monkey chatter' of thought and so reveal pure consciousness, which is held to be the ground of being. But the reasons for practising meditation today are no longer only those associated with mysticism or the occult. Recent studies at Western medical centres have shown clearly that meditation induces marked physiological and psychological changes associated with rest and relaxation of a transforming quality. Investigations into the physiology of meditation show that it reduces stress, reduces the breathing rate and the metabolic rate (oxygen consumption), lowers blood pressure in cases where the level is too high, and reduces the concentration of lactate in the blood. EEG equipment shows that deep meditation produces orderly brain patterns of beta and theta waves that are distinct from the patterns observed during drowsiness, sleep and hypnosis. These physiological effects are those that are associated with very deep rest and relaxation.

The psychological effects of meditation are also related to psychophysical poise and relaxation. Studies show that meditation reduces depression and neuroticism and also reduces the craving for drugs, cigarettes and alcohol. Furthermore, with repeated exposure to the deep thought-free awareness of meditation everyday living becomes more open, anxiety free, spontaneous, healthful, creative and rewarding in interpersonal relationships.

Traditionally, the Yoga taught in the present volume is viewed as a preparation for the Yoga of meditation. In the light of modern knowledge on the physiological and psychological effects of Eastern-style meditation this integral association of the two kinds of Yoga practice is justified more than ever. The Yoga of meditation intensifies and completes the transformation in the quality of living established by the Yoga of breath controls and posture.

Bibliography

Works on Hatha Yoga

1. Acharya, Pundit, *Breath Is Life*, Prana Press, New York, 1939.
2. Aiyengar, Srinivasa, (tr.), *Hatha Yoga Pradipika*, Tkaram Tastya, Bombay, 1933.
3. Alain, *Yoga for Perfect Health*, Thorsons, 1957.
4. Atkinson, W., *Hatha Yoga*, Yogi Publishing Society, Chicago, 1904.
   Avalon, Arthur, see Woodroffe, Sir John.
5. Bahm, Archie J., *Yoga for Business Executives*, Stanley Paul, 1967.
6. Behanan, Kovoor Y., *Yoga: A Scientific Evaluation*, Macmillan, New York, 1937; Dover, New York, 1959.
7. Bernard, Theos, *Hatha Yoga*, Columbia University Press, New York, 1944; Rider, London, 1950.
8. Bragdon, Claude, *Yoga For You*, Alfred A. Knopf, New York, 1943.
9. Brahmachari, Dhirendra, *Yogasana Vijnana*, Asia Publishing House, 1970.
10. Brena, S. F., *Yoga and Medicine*, Julian Press, New York, 1972.
11. Briggs, G. W., *Gorakhnath and the Kanphata Yogis*, Oxford University Press, 1938.
12. Carr, Rachel, *Yoga For All Ages*, Simon and Schuster, New York, 1972.
13. Chrishop, E. D., *Keep Young Through Yoga*, Health For All, 1956.
14. Danielou, Alain, *Yoga: the Method of Reintegration*, University Books, New York, 1949; Johnson Publications, London, 1949.
15. Day, Harvey, *Study and Practice of Yoga*, Thorsons, 1953.
16. Day, Harvey, *Practical Yoga for the Business Man*, Pelham Books, 1970; Drake Publishers, New York, 1970.
17. Day, Harvey, *Yoga Illustrated Dictionary*, Kaye and Ward, 1971.
18. Dechanet, J. M., O.S.B., *Yoga in Ten Lessons*, Harper, New York, 1965; Burns and Oates, London, 1965.
    Devi, Indra, see Strakaty, Eugenie.
19. Dey, P., *Yogic System of Exercise*, Luzac, 1934.
20. Dukes, Sir Paul, *The Yoga of Health, Youth, and Joy*, Cassell, 1960.
21. Garde, R. V., *Principles and Practice of Yoga Therapy*, Taraporevala, Bombay, 1972.
22. Garrison, O. V., *Tantra: the Yoga of Sex*, Julian Press, New York, 1965.
    Gheranda Samhita, see Vasu, Sris Chandra.
23. Goswami, S. S., *Hatha Yoga*, Fowler, 1963.
24. Gould, J., *Yoga for Heatlh and Beauty*, Thorsons, 1969.
25. Gunaji, N. V., *Scientific and Efficient Breathing*, N. V. Gunaji, Bombay, 1948.
26. Gupta, Yogi, *Yoga and Long Life*, Dodd Mead, Toronto, 1958; Y. Gupta, New York, 1965.
    Guyot, Felix, see Kerneiz, C.
    Hatha Yoga Pradipika, see Sinh, Pancham.
27. Hewitt, James, *Teach Yourself Yoga*, The English Universities Press, 1960; retitled *A Practical Guide to Yoga*, Funk and Wagnalls, New York, 1968.

28. Hewitt, James, *Yoga and You*, Anthony Gibbs, 1966; Tandem, 1967; Pyramid, New York, 1967.
29. Hittleman, R. L., *Be Young with Yoga*, Prentice-Hall, Englewood Cliffs, N.J., 1962; A. Thomas, Preston, 1963.
30. Hittleman, R. L., *Yoga for Physical Fitness*, Prentice-Hall, Englewood Cliffs, N.J.; A. Thomas, Preston, 1967.
31. Hittleman, R. L., *The Yoga Way to Figure and Facial Beauty*, Hawthorn Books, New York, 1969.
32. Hutchinson, Ronald, *Yoga a Way of Life*, Hamlyn, 1975.
33. Iyengar, B. K. S., *Light on Yoga*, Allen and Unwin, 1966.
34. Johns, June, with Mehr. S. Fardoonjhi, *Practical Yoga*, David and Charles, Newton Abbot, 1975.
35. Kerneiz, C. (Guyot, Felix), *Yoga: the Science of Health*, Dutton, New York, 1937; Rider, London, 1937.
36. Kiss, M., *Yoga for Young People*, Bobbs-Merrill, New York, 1971.
37. Krishnananda, R., *Mystery of Breath*, Para-vidya Centre, New York, 1940.
38. Kumar, N., *Aerobics and Yoga*, Whitmore, Philadelphia, 1973.
39. Krishna, Gopi, *Higher Consciousness*, Julian Press, New York, 1975.
40. Krishna, Gopi, *The Biological Basis of Religion and Genius*, New York Press, New York, 1971.
41. Krishna, Gopi, *The Secret of Yoga*, Harper, New York, 1972; Turnstone, London, 1973.
42. Kuvalayananda, Swami, *Yoga Mimansa Journals*, Lonavla, Bombay, 1924.
43. Kuvalayananda, Swami, *Pranayama*, Lonavla, Bombay, 1931.
44. Kuvalayananda, Swami, *Srimat Asanas*, Lonavla, Bombay, 1931.
45. Kuvalayananda, Swami, *Popular Yoga Asanas*, Prentice-Hall, Englewood Cliffs, N.J., 1972.
46. Lee-Richardson, J., *Manual of Yoga*, Foulsham, 1956.
47. Lee-Richardson, J., *Yoga Made Easy*, Prentice-Hall, Englewood Cliffs, N.J., 1961.
48. Liebers, A., *Relax with Yoga*, Oak Tree Press, 1960.
49. Louis-Frederick, *Yoga Asanas*, Thorsons, 1959.
50. Lysebeth, Andre van, *Yoga Self-Taught*, Harper, New York, 1972; Allen and Unwin, London, 1972.
51. Marwaha, B. S., *Health and Efficiency through Yoga Asanas*, Army Educational Publications, New Delhi, 1965.
52. Mia, T., *Get in Touch with Yourself through Yoga*, Prentice-Hall, Englewood Cliffs, N.J., 1972; Luscombe, London, 1975.
53. Mumford, J., *Psychosomatic Yoga*, Thorsons, 1962.
54. Murphet, H., *Yoga For Busy People*, Old Bourne Press, London, 1964; Soccer Associates, New Rochdale, N.Y., 1965.
55. Mazumar, S., *Yogic Exercises*, Longmans, 1954.
56. Narayananda, Swami, *Secrets of Prana, Pranayama, and Yoga-asanas*, N. K. Prasad, Rishikesh, 1959.
57. Oki, M., *Practical Yoga*, Japan Publications, Tokyo and New York, 1971.
58. Oman, J. C., *The Mystics, Ascetics, and Saints of India*, Unwin, London, 1899.

59. Phelan, N. C. and Volin, M., *Yoga For Women*, Harper, New York, 1963; Pelham, London, 1963.
60. Phelan, N. C. and Volin, M., *Yoga For Beauty*, London, 1965.
61. Phelan, N. C. and Volin, M., *Yoga Breathing*, Pelham, 1966.
62. Phelan, N. C. and Volin, M., *Sex and Yoga*, Harper, New York, 1967; Pelham, London, 1967.
63. Phelan, N. C. and Volin, M., *Growing up with Yoga*, Harper, New York, 1969; Pelham, London, 1969.
64. Pratinidhi, S. B. P., *The Ten-Point Way to Health*, Dent, 1938.
65. Rawls, E. S., *A Handbook of Yoga for Modern Living*, Parker, West Nyack, N.Y., 1966.
66. Rawls, E. S. and Diskin, E., *Yoga for Beauty and Health*, Horwitz, Sydney, 1969.
67. Rele, V. G., *The Mysterious Kundalini*, Taraporevala, Bombay, 1927.
68. Rele, V. G., *Yogic Asanas*, Taraporevala, Bombay, 1939.
69. Rieker, Hans-Ulrich (tr.), *The Yoga of Light: Hatha Yoga Pradipika, India's Classical Handbook*, Allen and Unwin, 1972.
70. Roy, A. T., *Nervous System of the Ancient Hindu*, Hazaribagh, 1930.
71. Ruchpaul, E., *Hatha Yoga*, Funk and Wagnalls, New York, 1970.
72. Saraswati, S., *Hatha Yoga*, Yoga Vedanta Forest University, Rishikesh, 1939.
73. Saraswati, S., *Yogic Home Exercises*, Taraporevala, Bombay, 1939; Kegan Paul, London, 1939.
74. Satchidananda, Swami, *Integral Hatha Yoga*, Holt, Rinehart, and Winston, New York, 1970.
75. Sinh, Pancham, (tr.), *Hatha Yoga Pradipika*, Lalit Mohan Basu, The Panini Office, Allahabad, 1915.
76. Sivananda, Swami, *Yoga Asanas*, Madras, 1934.
77. Sivananda, Swami, *Yogic Home Exercises*, Taraporevala, Bombay, 1944.
78. Sivananda, Swami, *Kundalini Yoga*, Divine Light Society, Rishikesh.
79. Sivananda, Swami and Vishnudevananda, Swami, *Practical Guide for Students of Yoga*, Divine Light Society, Hong Kong.
    Siva Samhita, see Vidyarnava, R. B. S. C.
80. Spring, C. and Goss, M. G., *Yoga For Today*, Holt, Rinehart and Winston, New York, 1959; A. Thomas, Preston, 1959.
81. Stearn, Jess, *Yoga, Youth, and Reincarnation*, Neville Spearman, 1966.
82. Strakaty, Eugenie (Indra Devi), *Forever Young, Forever Healthy*, Prentice-Hall, Englewood Cliffs, N.J., 1953; A. Thomas, Preston, 1955.
83. Strakaty, Eugenie, *Yoga for Americans*, Prentice-Hall, Englewood Cliffs, N.J., 1959; retitled *Yoga For You*, A. Thomas, Preston, 1960.
84. Strakaty, Eugenie, *Renew Your Life Through Yoga*, Prentice-Hall, Englewood Cliffs, N.J., 1963; Allen and Unwin, London, 1963.
85. Sundaram, S., *Yogic Physical Culture*, Bandalore, 1931.
86. Sunita, Y., *Pranayama Yoga*, West Midlands Press, Walsall, 1966.
87. Vasu, Sris Chandra, (tr.), *Gheranda Samhita*, Adyar, Madras, 1933.
88. Vidyarnava, Rai Bahadur Srisa Chandra, (tr.), *Siva Samhita*, Sudhindra Nath Basu, The Panini Office, Allahabad, 1923.

89. Vishnudevananda, Swami, *The Complete Illustrated Book of Yoga*, Julian Press, New York, 1960; Souvenir Press, London, 1961.
90. Vithaldas, Yogi, *The Yoga System of Health*, Faber, 1939; Greenberg, New York, 1950.
91. Wood, Ernest, *Yoga*, Penguin Books, 1959.
92. Woodroffe, Sir John (Arthur Avalon), *The Serpent Power*, Ganesh, Madras, 1918.
93. Woodroffe, Sir John, *Shakti and Shakta*, Ganesh, Madras, 1929.
94. Yesudian, S. R. and Haich, E., *Yoga and Health*, Allen and Unwin, 1966.
95. Yogendra, Shri, *Physical Education*, The Yoga Institute, Bombay, 1928.
96. Yogendra, Shri, *Yoga : Personal Hygiene*, The Yoga Institute, Bombay, 1943.
97. Yogendra, Sita Devi, *Yoga For Women*, The Yoga Institute, Bombay, 1943.
98. Young, F. R., *Yoga For Men Only*, Parker, West Nyack, N.Y., 1969.
99. Zorn, William, *Body Harmony : the easy Yoga exercise way*, Hawthorn, New York, 1971; retitled *The Easy Yoga Exercise Book*, Pelham, London, 1971.

General Works
100. *Asiatic Monthly Journal*, Madras, 1829. Included in H. H. Wilson, *A Sketch of the Religious Sects of the Hindus*, London, 1862; Calcutta, 1958.
101. Cannon, Alexander, *The Invisible Influence*, Rider, 1933; Acquarian Press, 1969.
102. Cooper, Kenneth H., M.D., *Aerobics*, Evans, New York, 1968.
103. David-Neel, Alexandra, *With Mystics and Magicians in Tibet*, John Lane, 1931.
104. Eliade, Mircea, *Images and Symbols*, Paris, 1952; Harvill Press, 1961.
105. Hewitt, James, *Techniques of Sex Fitness*, Universal, New York, 1969.
106. Honigberger, John Martin, 35 *Years in the East*, London, 1852.
107. Kimura, S., Ashiba, M. and Matsushima, I., 'Influence of the Air Lacking in Light Ions and the Effect of its Artificial Ionization Upon Human Beings in Occupied Rooms', Japanese Journal of Medical Science, 7 (1939).
108. Kotaka, S. and Kreuger, A. P., 'Studies on Air Ionized-Induced Growth Increase in Higher Plants', Advancing Frontiers of Plant Sciences, 20 (1967).
109. Kreuger, A. P., 'Preliminary Consideration of the Biological Significance of Air Ions', Scientia, 104 (Sept-Oct 1969). Included in Robert E. Ornstein (ed.), The Nature of Human Consciousness, Freeman, San Francisco, 1973.
110. Le Vay, David, *Teach Yourself Human Anatomy and Physiology*, The English Universities Press, 1972.
111. Maraini, Fosco, *Secret Tibet*, Bari, Italy, 1951; Hutchinson, 1952.
112. Maspero, Henri, 'Les Procedes de "nourrir le principe vital" dans la religion Taoiiste ancienne', Journal Asiatique, Paris, ccxxvii (1937). Included in Mircea Eliade, Yoga: Immortality and Freedom, Routledge and Kegan Paul, 1958.

113. Miller, Benjamin F. and Goode, Ruth, *Man and His Body*, Gollancz, 1961.
114. Muller, Max (tr.), *The Upanishads*, the Sacred Books of the East, vol. 1 1879 and vol. xv 1884, Clarendon Press, Oxford.
115. Ornstein, Robert E., *The Psychology of Consciousness*, Freeman, San Francisco, 1972.
116. Reich, Wilhelm, *The Discovery of the Orgone*, Noonday Press, New York, 1942.
117. *Strand Magazine*, vol. xiii, pages 176–180 (1897).
118. Tchijevsky, A. L., Transactions of the Central Laboratory Science Research Ionification, The Commune Publication House, Veronej, 1933.
119. Watts, Alan, *Cloud Hidden, Whereabouts Unknown: A Mountain Journal*, Cape, 1974.
120. Wood, Ernest, *The Occult Training of the Hindus*, Ganesh, Madras, 1931.